Interview Guide for Evaluating DSM-5-TR Psychiatric Disorders and the Mental Status Examination

Mark Zimmerman, M.D.

Professor of Psychiatry & Human Behavior
Brown University
Director, Outpatient Psychiatry & Partial Hospital Program
Rhode Island Hospital
Providence, Rhode Island

***P**sych **P**roducts **P**ress*
East Greenwich, RI

P.O. Box 228, East Greenwich, RI 02818

Printed in the United States of America.

ISBN: 978-0-9633821-2-2

To Caryn, Kyle, and Cali.

TABLE OF CONTENTS

Introduction 3
Components of the Psychiatric Evaluation 5
Beginning the Psychiatric Interview 6
Adult Disorders
Anorexia Nervosa 8
Binge Eating Disorder 9
Bulimia Nervosa 10
Alcohol Use Disorder 12
Drug Use Disorder 16
Gambling Disorder 22
Schizophrenia and Other Psychotic Disorders 24
Assessing Delusions and Hallucinations 28
Manic Episode 32
Hypomanic Episode 36
Major Depressive Disorder 40
Persistent Depressive Disorder. 44
Premenstrual Dysphoric Disorder 46
Panic Disorder 48
Agoraphobia 50
Social Anxiety Disorder (Social Phobia) 52
Specific Phobia 54
Generalized Anxiety Disorder 56
Posttraumatic Stress Disorder 58
Acute Stress Disorder 64
Prolonged Grief Disorder 68
Adjustment Disorder 71
Obsessive-Compulsive Disorder 72
Hoarding Disorder 74
Body Dysmorphic Disorder 76
Excoriation (Skin Picking) Disorder 78
Trichotillomania (Hair Pulling Disorder) 79
Intermittent Explosive Disorder 80
Illness Anxiety Disorder 82
Somatic Symptom Disorder 84
Attention Deficit Disorder (Adult) 85

Childhood Disorders
Attention Deficit Disorder (Child) 92
Conduct Disorder 98
Oppositional Defiant Disorder 102
Separation Anxiety Disorder 104
Personality Disorders
Paranoid Personality Disorder (PD) 108
Schizoid PD 110
Schizotypal PD 112
Borderline PD 116
Antisocial PD 120
Narcissistic PD 126
Histrionic PD 130
Obsessive-compulsive PD 133
Avoidant PD 136
Dependent PD 138
Mental Status Examination 140
Outline 141
Mini-Mental State Exam (Folstein). 143
Glossary of Terms 146
Current Psychosocial Functioning 152

INTRODUCTION

This book provides questions for evaluating psychiatric disorders.DSM-5-TR lists the disorders and their criteria, but it does not guide the beginner in inquiry for them. Students and clinicians in training are relatively unfamiliar with psychiatric diagnoses, and they cannot possibly remember all of the disorders and their corresponding diagnostic criteria within a short period of study. Moreover, it is often not obvious what questions to ask to determine the symptom's presence. How do you inquire for thought withdrawal, delusions of reference, panic attacks, obsessions, identity disturbance, mood instability, etc? Even more basic, how do you begin the interview?

The *Interview Guide* consists of questions for the most common DSM-5 diagnoses including the personality disorders. This book is not a standardized interview, to be started on page x and followed until page xx. Rather it is a quick reference to be used in the context of a clinical interview. If a patient complains of depression, the interviewer can turn to the section on major depression and assess the relevant symptoms. If there is a suggestion of excessive drug or alcohol use, the interviewer can refer to the long list of questions for diagnosing a drug or alcohol use disorder.

The book contains 9 sections. First, is a listing of the components of a complete psychiatric evaluation. This is followed by a brief section on how to begin a psychiatric interview. Sections 3, 4, and 5 include questions to assess the most common adult and childhood disorders and all of the personality disorders. Of note, the demarcation between Adult and Childhood disorders is not technically correct insofar as many of the Adult disorders can onset in childhood. It was tempting to label section 3 "Disorders Formerly Called Axis I Disorders" (to distinguish them from the personality disorders, which were placed on Axis II in DSM-III and DSM-IV), but this seemed too sarcastic. In section 6, I describe the mental status examination and provide a standardized outline for its charting and oral presentation. Also included is the mini-mental state exam which should be a part of every psychiatric evaluation. Section 7 is a glossary of commonly used psychiatric terms, and the final two sections include a brief psychosocial interview and a current psychosocial functioning assessment.

The book is organized by diagnosis. Listed in the box at the beginning of each section are the DSM-5-TR diagnostic rules—which and how many criteria must be present (inclusion criteria) and absent (exclusion criteria) for the diagnosis to be made. For most disorders, the initial questions in each section can be considered screening questions. If these screening questions are answered negatively, then it is reasonable to skip the remaining questions in the section.

The exception to the diagnosis-based organization is the section on the five psychotic disorders—schizophrenia, delusional disorder, schizoaffective disorder, schizophreniform disorder, and brief psychotic disorder. Questions to assess delusions and hallucinations are given in one section, and differential diagnosis is outlined and discussed in another.

The *Guide* should be used in conjunction with the DSM-5-TR manual. For most diagnoses covered in the *Guide*, the DSM-5-TR criteria (or a slight abbreviation of them) precede the relevant questions. However, the criteria are not included for the five psychotic disorders in the "Schizophrenia and Other Psychotic Disorders" section. Moreover, the DSM-5-TR manual includes lucid discussions of differential diagnosis.

Most criteria are assessed by several questions, and follow-ups to the initial questions are preceded by phrases typed in bold face such as **IF YES** or **IF NO**. This is a shorthand way of instructing the interviewer to ask additional questions. For example, **IF YES** means that the ensuing questions should be asked only if the response to the preceding one was yes.

Use of this guide does not guarantee competence. Interviewing involves more than the recitation of listed questions. With experience the clinician develops a style that generates a database for making diagnoses, as well as beginning a therapeutic relationship. Psychiatric diagnosis is not just based on responses to questions. It also relies on observation and evaluation of affect, behavior, and cognition (the ABC's of the mental status examination). Also, organic causes of symptoms must be ruled out. However, it is difficult to conduct a psychiatric interview if you do not know what questions to ask. That is the primary purpose of the *Interview Guide*.

Acknowledgement—Semi-structured diagnostic interviews have been widely used in psychiatric research during the past 40 years. I have been involved in developing some of these measures, and have been trained in others. The questions in the *Guide* derive, in part, from this experience. Because there are only a limited number of ways to ask about such symptoms as appetite change, sleep disturbance, etc., the questions will resemble the questions from these interviews, and they deserve acknowledgement. Specifically, had not the Schedule for Affective Disorders and Schizophrenia (SADS), Kiddie SADS, Structured Clinical Interview for DSM-IV, and Structured Interview for DSM-IV Personality Disorders not existed, then the present guide would not have been as rich and complete. Of course, the *Interview Guide* does not just include a listing of questions, but it also includes an overview and description of the mental status examination, a glossary of psychiatric terms, and a psychosocial history interview. Thus, the *Interview Guide* should help students and beginning clinicians perform a complete psychiatric evaluation.

COMPONENTS OF THE PSYCHIATRIC EVALUATION

Identifying data	(name, sex, age, race, marital status, source of history, reliability of patient as historian)
Chief complaint	(in patient's own words and in quotes)
History of present illness	
Past psychiatric history	
Past medical and surgical history	
Current medications	
Drug allergies	
Medical review of systems	
Substance use history	(See pages 12-21)
Family history	
Psychosocial history	(See pages 158-159)
Mental status exam	(See pages 146-151)
Physical exam	
Differential diagnosis	
Formulation	
Treatment plan	

BEGINNING THE PSYCHIATRIC INTERVIEW

The patient is likely to be nervous. Anxiety, which may be a symptom of their illness or due to their concern about speaking to a mental health professional, is the rule. The patient may be paranoid and suspicious of an unfamiliar doctor. They may also be angry because they are not there willingly. Perhaps they have been involuntarily committed, or perhaps a friend, family member, or boss strongly encouraged or coerced them to be evaluated. Thus, it is important to realize that an important purpose of the initial evaluation is to provide support and understanding to the patient, establish a trusting doctor-patient relationship, a by-product of which will be the information necessary to derive a diagnosis, formulation, and treatment plan. Of course, even the most experienced and skilled clinician cannot achieve this with all patients.

The evaluation should begin by introducing yourself. Refer to the patient by his/her name. Often it is helpful to tell the patient approximately how long the evaluation will take. The initial inquiry should be in a more open-ended, nonstructured manner. After an overview is obtained, more focused questions can be asked. Because most patients have usually spoken to a nurse or social worker before I interview them, I typically begin my evaluation:

> Hello Mr. Jones, I'm Dr. Zimmerman. I know you've already spoken to someone about what's been going on, and I know I'll be repeating some of the questions they already asked, but it's important and helpful for me to hear you tell your story. I would like to talk with you for about an hour to find out what has happened and how you've been feeling. .
>
> So tell me, what's been bothering you (going on)?
> How long has this been going on?
> What else has happened?
> You said these problems began_____. So, what's changed that you are coming for treatment now?

The information from these questions should help you determine which domains of psychopathology to explore in greater detail (i.e., which sections of the *Guide* to turn to). If the patient complains of depression, you should ask the questions about major depression and dysthymia (i.e., Persistent Depressive Disorder) on pages 40-46. If the patient described what sounds like an anxiety attack, you should turn to pages 48-49 for questions about Panic Disorder. And so on. The questions for the 10 personality disorders are on pages 114-145. Childhood disorders are covered on pages 98-112.

Adult Disorders

ANOREXIA NERVOSA

Inclusion: A-C
Exclusion: none

(A) Restriction of energy intake relative to requirements, leading to a significantly low body weight in the context of age, sex, developmental trajectory, and physical health. Significantly low body weight is defined as a weight that is less than minimally normal, or, for children and adolescents, less than minimally expected.

Has there ever been a time when people gave you a hard time about being too thin or losing too much weight?

Have you ever weighed much less than people thought you should?

IF YES TO EITHER QUESTION:
When did this occur? Is this still true?
What was the lowest you weighed?
How tall were you (at the time)?
What do you weigh now?

(B) Intense fear of gaining weight or of becoming fat, or persistent behavior that interferes with weight gain, even though at a significantly low weight.

During [TIME WHEN UNDERWEIGHT] were you very afraid of gaining weight or becoming fat?
IF NO: During this time, did you do anything to try and keep your weight low? **IF YES:** Describe.

(C) Disturbance in the way in which one's body weight or shape is experienced, undue influence of body weight or shape on self-evaluation, or persistent lack of recognition of the seriousness of the current low body weight.

During that time how did you think your body looked?
Did others say you were thin, but you thought you looked fat?
Did any part of your body feel fat? **IF YES:** Which part?
Did your weight or the shape of your body have a big effect on your opinion of yourself? **IF YES:** Tell me about that.
How much did you think about the health risks of weighing so little?
Did anyone tell you that it was not good for your health to be so thin?

BINGE EATING DISORDER

Inclusion: A-D
Exclusion: E

(A) Recurrent episode of binge eating as characterized by <u>both</u>:
1) Eating in discrete period of time (e.g., within any 2-hour period) an amount of food that is definitely larger than what most people would eat during a similar period of time under similar circumstances.
2) A sense of lack of control over eating during the episode (e.g., a feeling that one cannot stop eating or control what or how much one is eating).

1) Have you ever gone on eating binges when you ate abnormally large amounts of food over a short period of time?
   IF YES: What would you eat during a binge?
2) During a binge did you feel you lost control of your eating?

(B) The binge-eating episodes are associated with 3 or more of the following:

During these binges did you...
1) eat much more rapidly than normal?
2) eat until you felt uncomfortably full?
3) eat large amounts of food after you didn't feel physically hungry?
4) eat alone because you were embarrassed by how much you were eating?
5) feel disgusted with yourself, depressed, or very guilty after eating so much?

(C) Marked distress regarding binge eating.

How much were you bothered by the binge eating?

(D) The binge eating occurs, on average, at least once a week for 3 months.

At its most frequent, how often did you binge?
(For how long did you do this?)
(Did you ever binge at least once a week for 3 months?)

(E) <u>Exclude</u> the diagnosis if the symptoms occur exclusively during episodes of bulimia nervosa or anorexia nervosa.

BULIMIA NERVOSA

Inclusion: A-D
Exclusion: E

(A) Recurrent episodes of binge eating as characterized by both:
1) Eating in discrete period of time (e.g., within any 2-hour period) an amount of food that is definitely larger than what most people would eat during a similar period of time under similar circumstances.
2) A sense of lack of control over eating during the episode (e.g., a feeling that one cannot stop eating or control what or how much one is eating).

1) Have you ever gone on eating binges when you ate abnormally large amounts of food over a short period of time?
IF YES: What would you eat during a binge?

2) During a binge did you feel you lost control of your eating?

(B) Recurrent inappropriate compensatory behaviors in order to prevent weight gain, such as self-induced vomiting; misuse of laxatives, diuretics, or other medications; fasting; or excessive exercise.

To prevent gaining weight from the binge, would you sometimes…
…force yourself to vomit?
…go on very strict diets or fast afterwards?
…use laxatives or water pills?
…use diet pills?
…exercise excessively?
IF YES TO ANY: Describe what that was like.

(C) The binge eating and inappropriate compensatory behaviors both occur, on average, at least once per week for 3 months.

At its most frequent, how often did you binge?
(For how long did you do this?)
(Did you ever binge at least once a week for 3 months?)

How often did you [COMPENSATORY BEHAVIOR]?
(Did you ever [COMPENSATORY BEHAVIOR] at least once a week for 3 months?)

(D) Self-evaluation is unduly influenced by body shape and weight.

Did your weight or the shape of your body have a big effect on your opinion of yourself?

IF YES: Tell me about that.

(E) <u>Exclude</u> the diagnosis if the symptoms occur exclusively during episodes of anorexia nervosa.

IF ANOREXIC: Did you also binge and [COMPENSATORY BEHAVIOR] when you weren't underweight like you were when you were [AGE]?

ALCOHOL USE DISORDER

Inclusion: at least 2 criteria
Exclusion: none

Screening Questions

Now I'm going to ask you some questions about your use of alcohol.

What are your drinking habits like?
(How many times per week do you drink?)
(When you drink how many drinks do you have?)

Was there ever a time in your life when you drank too much?
IF YES: When was that? (How old were you?)

Has anyone in your family ever said that you were an excessive drinker?

Have friends, a doctor, or anyone else ever said that you drink too much?

Have you ever been concerned or upset about your drinking?

Has alcohol ever caused problems for you?
IF YES: What kind of problems?
How old were you when you had these problems?

A problematic pattern of alcohol use leading to clinically significant impairment or distress, as manifested by 2 or more of the following occurring within a 12-month period.

(1) Alcohol is often taken in larger amounts or over a longer period than was intended.

When you drank, did you often drink more than you had planned?

When you drank, did you often drink for more time than you had planned?

(2) There is a persistent desire or unsuccessful efforts to cut down or control alcohol use.

Did you frequently think about cutting down or stopping drinking?
IF YES: How much did you think about that?
For how long did you think about that? (A week? Months?)

At times, did you try to cut down or stop but couldn't?
IF NO: For example, some people try to control their drinking by promising not to begin before a certain time or not to drink alone. Did you ever do things like that?
IF YES: How often did you try to cut back or stop completely?

(3) A great deal of time is spent in activities necessary to obtain alcohol, use alcohol, or recover from its effects.

Did you spend a lot of time doing things and planning ways to get alcohol? **IF YES:** Was this the number one thing on your mind?

How much time did you spend drinking?

How often were you intoxicated?

Did you spend a lot of time recovering from hangovers?

(4) Craving, or a strong desire or urge to use alcohol.

Have you ever experienced cravings or strong urges for alcohol?
IF YES: Describe what that was like.

(5) Recurrent alcohol use resulting in a failure to fulfill major role obligations at work, school, or home.

Because of drinking, how often did you…
…come late to, or miss, work (or school)?
…have trouble at work (or school)?
…fail classes?
…get fired (or suspended or expelled from school)?
…not take care of children?
…not cook, clean the house, or go grocery shopping?

(6) Continued alcohol use despite having persistent or recurrent social or interpersonal problems caused or exacerbated by the effects of alcohol.

Because of drinking, did you…

…frequently have problems or arguments with friends or family?
…spend less time with family or friends?
…get separated or divorced?
…get into physical fights?
…get violent?

IF YES TO ANY: Did you still drink despite these problems?

(7) Important social, occupational, or recreational activities are given up or reduced because of alcohol use.

Did you spend so much of your time drinking that you…

…missed a lot of time from work?
…spent less time with family or friends?
…gave up some hobbies or other interests?

IF YES TO ANY: Tell me about that.

(8) Recurrent alcohol use in situations in which it is physically hazardous.

Did you drive while intoxicated (or had too much to drink)?
IF YES: How often?

Did you ever drink and then do something that was potentially physically dangerous (e.g., operate machinery)? **IF YES:** How often?

(9) Alcohol use is continued despite knowledge of having a persistent or recurrent physical or psychological problem that is likely to have been caused or exacerbated by the alcohol.

Did drinking cause medical or physical problems?
Did it cause anxiety, depression, or any other psychological problem?
Did you ever have blackouts (i.e., you did not remember what happened to you while you were drinking)?

IF YES TO ANY: Like what?
Did you keep drinking anyway?

(10) Tolerance, as defined by <u>either</u> of the following:
1. A need for a markedly increased amount of alcohol to achieve intoxication or desired effect.
2. A markedly diminished effect with continued use of the same amount of alcohol.

1. Over time did you need to drink a lot more to get the same effect as before? **IF YES:** How much more?

2. Did you develop a tolerance to alcohol so that the same amount as previously did not have the same effect?

(11) Withdrawal, as manifested by <u>either</u> of the following:
1. Within several hours to a few days after cessation or reduction of heavy and prolonged alcohol use, the person experienced at least 2 characteristic symptoms of withdrawal.
2. Alcohol (or closely related substance such as benzodiazepine) is taken to relieve or avoid withdrawal symptoms.

1. Did you experience any of the following withdrawal symptoms when you quit or cut down your drinking:
   1) Heart racing or sweating
   2) Hand tremor
   3) Sleep problems
   4) Nausea or vomiting
   5) Hallucinations
   6) Feeling fidgety, restless, or agitated
   7) Anxiety or nervousness
   8) Seizures

   IF YES TO ANY: How soon after you quit or cut down did the [SYMPTOM] begin?

2. Would you drink or take anything else to stop the withdrawal symptoms, or to prevent them from coming on? (Did you drink in the morning to keep withdrawal symptoms from coming on?)

DRUG USE DISORDER

Inclusion: at least 2 criteria
Exclusion: none

Screening Questions

Street Drugs

Have you ever used any street drugs?
IF YES: What did you use? How frequently?

IF USED LESS THAN 10 TIMES IN LIFE, SKIP TO SCREENING QUESTIONS REGARDING PRESCRIBED MEDICINES

Was there ever a time in your life when you think you used drugs too much?
IF YES: When was that? (How old were you?)
Has anyone in your family ever said that you used drugs too much?
Have friends, a doctor, or anyone else ever said that you used drugs too much?
Have you ever been concerned or upset about your drug use?
Has drug use ever caused problems for you?
IF YES: What kind of problems?
How old were you when you had these problems?

Prescribed Medication

Have you ever used sleeping pills, tranquilizers, weight loss medicines, or painkillers?
IF YES: How long did you take [DRUG]?
Did you get hooked or addicted to it?
Did you ever take much more than was prescribed?

If all of the above questions are ANSWERED NO, the diagnosis of drug use disorder is unlikely.

A problematic pattern of drug use leading to clinically significant impairment or distress, as manifested by two or more of the following, occurring within a 12-month period.

(1) Drug is often taken in larger amounts or over a longer period than was intended.

When you used [DRUG], did you often use more than you had planned?

When you used [DRUG], did you often use it for a longer period of time than you had planned?

(2) There is a persistent desire or unsuccessful efforts to cut down or control drug use.

Did you frequently think about cutting down or stopping your use of [DRUG]?

IF YES: How much did you think about that?
For how long did you think about that? (A week? Months?)

At times, did you try to cut down or stop but couldn't?

IF NO: For example, some people try to control their drug use by promising not to begin before a certain time or not to use alone. Did you ever do things like that?

IF YES: How often did you try to cut back or stop completely?

(3) A great deal of time is spent in activities necessary to obtain drug, use drug, or recover from its effects.

Did you spend a lot of time doing things and planning ways to get drugs? **IF YES:** Was this the number one thing on your mind?

How much time did you spend using?

How often were you high?

Did you spend a lot of time recovering from using [DRUG]?

(4) Craving or strong desire or urge to use drug.

Have you ever experienced cravings or strong urges to take [DRUG]?
IF YES: Describe what that was like.

(5) Recurrent drug use resulting in a failure to fulfill major role obligations at work, school, or home.

Because of your [DRUG] use, how often did you…
…come late to, or miss, work (or school)?
…have trouble at work (or school)?
…fail classes?
…get fired (or suspended or expelled from school)?
…not take care of children?
…not cook, clean the house, or go grocery shopping?

(6) Continued drug use despite having persistent or recurrent social or interpersonal problems caused or exacerbated by the effects of the drug.

Because of your [DRUG] use, did you…
…frequently have problems or arguments with friends or family?
…spend less time with family or friends?
…get separated or divorced?
…get into physical fights?
…get violent?
IF YES TO ANY: Did you still use despite these problems?

(7) Important social, occupational, or recreational activities are given up or reduced because of drug use.

Did you spend so much of your time using/getting high that you…
…missed a lot of time from work?
…spent less time with family or friends?
…gave up some hobbies or other interests?
IF YES TO ANY: Tell me about that.

(8) Recurrent drug use in situations in which it is physically hazardous.

Did you drive while high on drugs? **IF YES:** How often?
Did you ever use drugs and then do something that was potentially physically dangerous (e.g., operate machinery)? **IF YES:** How often?

(9) Drug use is continued despite knowledge of having a persistent or recurrent physical or psychological problem that is likely to have been caused or exacerbated by the drug.

Did using [DRUG] cause medical or physical problems?
Did it cause anxiety, depression, or any other psychological problem?
IF YES TO EITHER: Like what?
Did you keep using anyway?

(10) Tolerance, as defined by <u>either</u> of the following:

1. **A need for a markedly increased amount of drug to achieve intoxication or desired effect.**
2. **Markedly diminished effect with continued use of the same amount of drug.**

1. Over time did you need to use a lot more [DRUG] to get the same effect as before? **IF YES:** How much more?

2. Did you develop a tolerance to [DRUG] so that the same amount as previously did not have the same effect?

NOTE: Criterion 11 refers to withdrawal from substances. Withdrawal symptoms vary according to the class of substance. On the following 2 pages questions are separately listed to determine withdrawal from 4 classes of substances—-cannabis, opioids, sedatives, and stimulants. Below, I first list the general criteria for withdrawal.

(11) Withdrawal, as manifested by <u>either</u> of the following:

1. **The characteristic withdrawal syndrome for the substance.**
2. **The same (or closely related) substance is taken to relieve or avoid withdrawal symptoms.**

(11) <u>Cannabis withdrawal</u> as manifested by <u>either</u> of the following:

1. Within a week after cessation of heavy and prolonged cannabis use (i.e., usually daily use or almost daily use for at least a few months; however, withdrawal symptoms can occur with less frequent but chronic use) at least 3 characteristic symptoms of withdrawal; or

2. The same (or closely related) substance is taken to relieve or avoid withdrawal symptoms.

1. Did you experience any of the following withdrawal symptoms within a week after you quit using [DRUG]?
   1) Irritable mood, anger outbursts, or violent episodes
   2) Nervousness or anxiety
   3) Insomnia or disturbing dreams
   4) Decreased appetite or weight loss
   5) Restlessness
   6) Depressed mood
   7) Physical symptoms such as stomach pain, shakiness, tremulousness, sweating, fever, chills, or headache.
2. Would you use [DRUG] to stop the withdrawal symptoms, or to prevent them from coming on?

(11) <u>Opioid withdrawal</u> as manifested by <u>either</u> of the following:

1. Within several minutes to a few days after cessation or reduction of heavy and prolonged opioid use (several weeks or longer), or administration of an opioid antagonist, at least 3 characteristic symptoms of withdrawal; or

2. The same (or closely related) substance is taken to relieve or avoid withdrawal symptoms.

1. Did you experience any of the following withdrawal symptoms soon after you quit or cut down your use of [DRUG] (or [OPIOID ANTAGONIST] was given to you)?
   1) Depressed or irritable mood
   2) Nausea or vomiting
   3) Muscle aches
   4) Teary eyes or runny nose
   5) Dilated pupils, goose bumps, or sweating
   6) Diarrhea
   7) Yawning
   8) Fever
   9) Decreased sleep
2. Would you use [DRUG] to stop the withdrawal symptoms, or prevent them from coming on?

(11) <u>Sedative/hypnotic withdrawal</u> as manifested by <u>either:</u>

1. Within several hours to a few days after cessation or reduction of prolonged sedative/hypnotic use, the person experienced at least 2 characteristic symptoms of withdrawal; or

2. The same (or closely related) substance is taken to relieve or avoid withdrawal symptoms.

1. Did you experience any of the following withdrawal symptoms soon after you quit or cut down your use of [DRUG]?
    1) Heart racing or sweating
    2) Hand tremor
    3) Sleep problems
    4) Nausea or vomiting
    5) Hallucinations or illusions
    6) Feeling fidgety, restless, or agitated
    7) Anxiety or nervousness
    8) Seizures
2. Would you take anything, or drink alcohol, to stop withdrawal symptoms, or to prevent them from coming on?

(11) <u>Stimulant withdrawal</u> as manifested by <u>either</u> of the following:

1. Within several hours to a few days after cessation or reduction of prolonged stimulant use, the person experienced dysphoric mood (item 1), and at least 2 other characteristic symptoms of withdrawal; or

2. The same (or closely related) substance is taken to relieve or avoid withdrawal symptoms.

1. Did you experience any of the following withdrawal symptoms soon after you quit or cut down your use of [DRUG]?
    1) Depressed or irritable mood
    2) Fatigue
    3) Vivid, unpleasant dreams
    4) Increased or decreased sleep
    5) Increased appetite
    6) Feeling fidgety, restless, or agitated, or the opposite, feeling slowed down like you were stuck in mud.
2. Would you use [DRUG] to stop withdrawal symptoms, or to prevent them from coming on?

GAMBLING DISORDER

Inclusion: at least 4 from A
Exclusion: B

Screening Questions

Did you ever gamble?

IF YES: When in your life did you gamble the most?
How long did that last? How often did you gamble?
How much were you betting?

Did you ever think that you had a problem with gambling?
Has anyone else ever thought that you have a gambling problem?
(How often do you gamble now?) (How much money are you gambling?)

A. Persistent and recurrent problematic gambling behavior leading to clinically significant impairment or distress, as indicated by 4 (or more) of the following in a 12-month period.

(A1) Needs to gamble with increasing amounts of money in order to achieve the desired excitement.

Have you found that over time you needed to increase the size or number of your bets to get a feeling of excitement? (Describe.)

(A2) Is restless or irritable when attempting to cut down or stop gambling.

Do you get restless or irritable when you try to cut down or stop gambling?

(A3) Has made repeated unsuccessful efforts to control, cut back or stop gambling.

How often have you tried to control, cut down, or stop gambling?

(A4) Is often preoccupied with gambling (e.g., persistent thoughts of reliving past gambling experiences, handicapping or planning the next venture, or thinking of ways to get money with which to gamble).

How much do you think about gambling?
Do you think a lot about how to get gambling money?
Do you spend a lot of time planning your next gambling trip?

(A5) Often gambles when feeling distressed (e.g., helpless, guilty, anxious, depressed).

Do you gamble in order to forget about your problems?
IF YES: Tell me about that.

Do you gamble in order to improve your mood?
IF YES: Tell me about that.

(A6) After losing money gambling, often returns another day to get even ("chasing" one's losses).

After losing money gambling, do you often go back another day to get even? **IF YES:** How often does that occur?

(A7) Lies to conceal the extent of involvement with gambling.

Have you ever lied to friends, family members, or others to hide the extent of your gambling? **IF YES:** Tell me about that.

(A8) Has jeopardized or lost a significant relationship, job, or educational or career opportunity because of gambling.

What effect has gambling had on your life?
Did you ever lose or almost lose a job?
Did you have to leave school?
Did you ever lose or almost lose an important relationship because of gambling?

(A9) Relies on others to provide money to relieve desperate financial situations caused by gambling.

Did you ever need other people to bail you out financially because of your gambling debts?

(B) The gambling behavior is not better accounted for by a Manic Episode.

Just before this began, were you feeling good, "high," excited, or hyper that other people thought that you were not your normal self? (Did anyone say you were manic?)

SCHIZOPHRENIA AND OTHER PSYCHOTIC DISORDERS

The diagnostic criteria for schizophrenia are complex and involve 1) inquiry for delusions and hallucinations, 2) inquiry for manic and depressive syndromes, and if these have been present, then determining whether they are brief relative to the duration of illness, 3) inquiry for the duration of the active psychotic symptom phase, as well as the residual and prodromal illness phases, 4) inquiry to determine deterioration in level of functioning, and 5) observation of affective, behavioral, and cognitive signs of illness.

The questions for detecting delusions and hallucinations are listed on pages 28-31. Questions regarding manic and depressive syndromes can be found on pages 32-35 and 40-43, respectively. Many of the prodromal/residual phase symptoms are similar to the schizotypal personality disorder criteria, and the relevant questions are on pages 118-121.

The user of this guide should refer to the DSM-5-TR manual to fully appreciate the differences between schizophrenia, delusional disorder, schizophreniform disorder, brief psychotic disorder and schizoaffective disorder. The common thread to these disorders is the presence of psychosis. The specific delusions and hallucinations are defined in the glossary. Unlike the other sections of this guide, the questions do not follow the DSM-5-TR diagnostic algorithms. Instead, I briefly summarize the salient features of these disorders, and then highlight differential diagnosis considerations for five pairs of disorders.

Schizophrenia is generally a chronic illness beginning before the age of 25 in which the individual does not return to his or her premorbid level of functioning. Prominent hallucinations or delusions are usually present. The person must be ill at least six months, though they need not be actively psychotic all of the time. Three phases of the illness are defined. The prodrome phase includes attenuated forms of active phase symptoms (e.g., odd beliefs, ideas of reference, unusual perceptual experiences), negative symptoms, and/or a deterioration in function prior to the onset of the active psychotic phase. The active phase symptoms (delusions, hallucinations, disorganized speech, grossly disorganized behavior, or negative symptoms such as avolition and flat affect) must be present for at least one month. The residual phase follows the active phase. The features of the residual and prodromal phases include functional impairment, and abnormalities in affect, cognition, and communication. If a manic or depressive syndrome occurs, it lasts for less than half the duration of the active and residual phases of the illness.

The DSM-5-TR definition of schizophrenia has 5 criteria. Criterion A, or the active phase of illness, requires the presence of two of the following features for at least one month (and at least 1 of these must be from the first 3 items): delusions, hallucinations, disorganized speech, grossly disorganized or catatonic behavior, and negative symptoms. Criterion B refers to social or occupational impairment, and Criterion C refers to the six-month duration of disturbance. Criteria D and E exclude the diagnosis if there is significant mood disorder pathology, or if the disturbance is due to the effects of street drugs, medication, or medical illness.

Delusional Disorder is also usually a chronic illness. The delusions last at least a month and usually involve situations that can occur in real life such as infidelity, being followed, or illness. If hallucinations are present they are not prominent and are related to the delusion. Functional impairment is linked to the delusional system. Often functioning is not markedly and pervasively impaired as it is in schizophrenia. If a manic or depressive syndrome occurs, its duration is brief relative to the duration of the delusion.

Brief Psychotic Disorder requires the presence of one or more of the following for at least one day but less than a month: delusions, hallucinations, disorganized speech, or grossly disorganized or catatonic behavior. Onset is usually sudden, impairment can be severe during the episode, but the individual returns to his or her normal self.

Schizophreniform Disorder lasts at least one month, but less than six months, and is characterized by delusions, prominent hallucinations, or the other active phase features of schizophrenia. Thus, Criterion A of schizophrenia is met except for the duration of the episode. A manic or depressive syndrome, if present, is present for only a minority of the duration of the psychotic symptoms. Thus, the criteria are similar to those of schizophrenia except the illness duration is less than six months, and there is no social or occupational impairment requirement. When the symptoms are current, and the episode duration is less than 6 months, the diagnosis should be qualified as provisional because it is not yet clear if the patient will meet the criteria for schizophrenia.

Schizoaffective Disorder is diagnosed when the patient has the characteristic features of the active phase of schizophrenia, but the duration of the manic or depressive syndrome is present for the majority of the duration of the active and residual phases of the illness. However, for at least two weeks the individual has delusions or hallucinations but not prominent mood symptoms (and this excludes the diagnosis of a mood disorder with psychotic features).

DIFFERENTIATING PSYCHOTIC DISORDERS

1. **Schizophrenia vs. Delusional Disorder**: In delusional disorder, the content of the delusions involves events that may actually occur to some people in real life (e.g., being followed by the FBI, having cancer, becoming a famous entertainer or author, being poisoned etc.). Bizarre delusions such as thought broadcasting and delusions of control, and prominent hallucinations, only occur in schizophrenia. Hallucinations can occur in individuals with delusional disorder; however, they are not prominent and are related to the delusional theme. Similarly, disorganized speech, grossly disorganized or catatonic behavior, and negative symptoms are usually absent in delusional disorder. Thus, criterion A of schizophrenia is not present. Nonbizarre delusions can occur in schizophrenia; however, they are not the only psychotic symptom. The individual with schizophrenia additionally experiences either prominent hallucinations, or markedly disturbed affect, thought processes, or behavior. The impairment associated with delusional disorder is usually circumscribed, whereas the impairment associated with schizophrenia is more global.

2. **Schizophrenia vs. Schizoaffective Disorder**: The psychotic symptoms are the same. In schizoaffective disorder a manic or depressive episode must be present, and the mood syndrome has been present for the majority of the time. However, to be diagnosed with schizoaffective disorder there must be at least two weeks in which the delusions or hallucinations are present but prominent mood symptoms are not.

3. **Schizoaffective Disorder vs. Mood Disorder with Psychotic Features**: In a psychotic mood disorder, there are no periods (or only very brief ones) characterized by psychosis but without prominent mood symptoms. You cannot rely on the content and type of psychotic symptoms, or the number and severity of mood symptoms, to distinguish these two disorders. Rather, the distinguishing factor is whether or not the psychotic and mood symptoms overlap in time.

4. **Schizophrenia vs. Schizophreniform Disorder**: The symptom inclusion criteria are the same. The primary difference is that schizophrenia lasts for more than six months (including the prodromal, active and residual phases), whereas in schizophreniform disorder the pathology (i.e., all three phases) has lasted less than six months.

5. **Schizophreniform Disorder vs. Brief Psychotic Disorder**: Both refer to psychotic disorders of brief duration. The psychotic symptom inclusion criteria are similar, but not identical. The psychosis inclusion criteria are broader for brief psychotic disorder (any one of: delusions, hallucinations, disorganized speech) versus criterion A of schizophrenia which requires at least two of five features. Schizophreniform disorder lasts at least a month, whereas brief psychotic disorder lasts less than a month.

ASSESSING DELUSIONS AND HALLUCINATIONS

DELUSION OF REFERENCE

When watching TV, listening to the radio, or reading the paper, do you notice that they are referring to you, or that there are special messages intended specifically for you?

IF YES: What have you noticed?

Does it seem like strangers on the street are taking special notice of you, or talking about you?

IF YES: Is it a feeling you have, or are you pretty sure that they are talking about/referring to you?

IF PRETTY SURE: How do you know?

Do things seem especially arranged for you?

IF YES: In what way?

DELUSION OF PERSECUTION

Is anybody against you, following you, giving you a hard time, or trying to hurt you?

IF YES: Tell me about that.

Do you feel like there's a plot to hurt you?

IF YES: Who's involved? Why would they want to hurt you?

THOUGHT BROADCASTING

Do you ever think of something so strongly that people could hear your thoughts?

IF YES: So, people can hear what you are thinking even when you're not talking?
How do you know?

DELUSION OF MIND READING

Are people able to read your mind and know what you're thinking?

IF YES: How can they do this?
Can anyone do it, or just some people? Who?
Do they literally read your thoughts, or do they read your facial expression to know what you're thinking?

THOUGHT WITHDRAWAL

Are your thoughts ever taken out of your head?

IF DOESN'T UNDERSTAND QUESTION:

Does someone or some force reach into your head and remove or steal your thoughts?

IF YES TO EITHER QUESTION:

Tell me about it.

THOUGHT INSERTION

Are there ever thoughts in your head that have been put in there from the outside?

IF YES: Tell me about it.

(I'm not referring to talking to someone who makes a suggestion or gives you advice. Instead, I'm referring to thoughts getting inserted into your head from the outside. Does this ever happen?)

DELUSION OF GUILT

(Also see Major Depression section, page 40.)

Do you think you've done something terrible and deserve to be punished?

IF YES: I know it will be hard to talk about, but what do you feel so guilty about?

Do you blame yourself for bad things going on in the world like starvation, wars, crime, etc.?

DELUSION OF GRANDIOSITY

(See Mania section, page 32.)

DELUSION OF CONTROL

Do you ever get the feeling that you're being controlled by some force or power from the outside?

IF YES: What's that like?
At times, does it seem like you're not in control of your body, almost like you're a puppet and something from the outside pulls the strings?

IF YES: If I asked you to raise your hand or stand up now, would you be able to do it?

IF NO: Why is that?

IF YES: So, you're in control of your actions?
Are you always in control?

SOMATIC DELUSION

Are you concerned that you have a serious physical illness that a doctor hasn't found, or that something is wrong with your body?

IF YES: What do you think is wrong?
Why do you think that?
Are you sure?

****
HALLUCINATIONS
****

VISUAL HALLUCINATIONS

Have you seen visions or other things that other people didn't see?

IF YES: What did you see?
What time of day did this occur?
How long ago did it start?
Do you see it every day?
How often do you see it?

AUDITORY HALLUCINATIONS

Have you heard noises, or sounds, or voices that other people didn't hear?

IF YES: What did you hear?

Do the voices seem to come from inside or outside your heard? **IF INSIDE:** But you hear it with your ears?

How many voices do you hear?

Are they male or female? Do you recognize them?

Do you ever hear two or more voices talking to each other?

Do the voices ever talk about what you're doing or thinking?

IF YES: Do they ever keep up a running commentary on what you're doing or thinking just like a sports announcer describes a ball game?

How long ago did the voices start?

Do you hear them every day?

How often during the day do you hear them?

Do they influence your behavior?

Do they tell you to do things?

TACTILE HALLUCINATIONS

Do you ever notice strange sensations in your body or on your skin?

Do you ever feel something creeping or crawling on your body, or something push or punch you but no one is there?

IF YES: Like what?

When did it happen the first time?

How often has it happened?

OLFACTORY AND GUSTATORY HALLUCINATIONS

What about smells that other people don't notice, or strange tastes in your mouth?

IF YES: Like what?

When did it happen the first time?

How often has it happened?

Are they associated with any other physical symptoms like an upset stomach, numbness, tingling, or brief memory loss?

IF YES: Tell me about that.

MANIC EPISODE

Inclusion: A, at least 3 or 4 from B, C
Exclusion: D,E

(A) A distinct period of abnormally and persistently elevated, expansive, or irritable mood, and abnormally and persistently increased goal directed activity or energy, lasting at least one week. and present most of the day nearly every day (or any duration if hospitalization is necessary).

Have there been times lasting at least several days when you felt high, on top of the world, euphoric, or overly cheery?
Have you had periods when you are more energetic or active than usual?

IF YES:

Describe what that was like.
How many periods like this have you had?
Does anything cause this? (Were you using any drugs?)
How is this different than a normal good mood?
How long do these periods typically last? (How long was the longest?)
Is your mood/energy/activity elevated almost all day long?

IF NO:

What about a period lasting several days when you were unusually irritable and quick to argue or fight?

IF YES:

Describe what that is like. (Does your energy increase?)
How many periods like this have you had?
Does your energy level seem higher during these times? (Are you more active?)
Does anything cause the irritable mood? (Substance use?)
How long do these periods typically last? (How long was the longest?)
During these periods do you feel irritable almost all day?

(Were you hospitalized for any of these periods?)

Now I'm going to ask about some other things that may have occurred at the same time you were feeling [MOOD STATE].

B. During the period of mood disturbance and increased energy or activity, 3 or more of the following symptoms (4 if the mood is only irritable) are present to a significant degree, and represent a noticeable change from usual behavior.

(B1) Inflated self-esteem or grandiosity.

What was your self-esteem like during this time?
Did you feel more self-confident than usual?
Did you feel like you had special talents, abilities, or powers?
IF YES: Like what?

When some people feel [MANIC MOOD] they may think they're going to become famous or do great things. Did you have any thoughts like that? **IF YES:** Like what?

(B2) Decreased need for sleep (e.g., feels rested after only 3 hours of sleep).

During this time how did you sleep?
Did you need less sleep than usual to feel rested?
IF YES: How many hours were you able to get by on?

(B3) More talkative than usual or pressure to keep talking.

Were you more talkative than usual?
Did you talk on and on so that it was hard for others to get a word in?
Did you feel a pressure to talk constantly?
Did you talk faster than you normally do?
IF YES: Did you talk so fast that it was hard to understand you?

(B4) Flight of ideas or subjective experience that thoughts are racing.

During this time did it feel like your thoughts were going very fast and racing through your mind?

(B5) Distractibility (i.e., attention too easily drawn to unimportant or irrelevant external stimuli) as reported or observed.

Were you easily distracted so that any little thing could get you off track?
IF YES: What was that like?

(B6) Increase in goal-directed activity (either socially, at work or school, or sexually) or psychomotor agitation (i.e., purposeless non-goal directed activity).

Were you more active than usual? For example, did you do more chores around the house?

Were you so energetic that instead of sleeping you did household chores or work throughout the night?

Did you start new projects or take on added responsibilities?

Did you work more?

Did you call friends more? Were you sexually more active than usual?

Did you feel physically restless so that it was hard to sit still?
Were you always moving or pacing back and forth?

IF YES TO ANY OF ABOVE: Tell me what you did.

(B7) Excessive involvement in activities that have a high potential for painful consequences (e.g., engaging in unrestricted buying sprees, sexual indiscretions, or foolish business investments).

Did you do anything that could have caused problems for you or your family? For example, when some people feel [MANIC MOOD] they go on spending sprees, write bad checks, invest money foolishly, or do things sexually that are unusual for them. Did you do anything like that? **IF YES:** Like what?

(C) The mood disturbance is sufficiently severe to cause marked impairment in social or occupational functioning or to necessitate hospitalization to prevent harm to self or others, or there are psychotic features.

What effect did this episode (these episodes) have on your life at the time it was going on?

Did it cause major problems in your job? School? Marriage? Social life? Relationships with friends or family?
IF YES TO ANY: What happened?

Did you get treatment? (Were you hospitalized?)

(D) <u>Exclude</u> the diagnosis if the symptoms are attributable to the direct physiological effects of a substance (e.g., a drug of abuse, a medication, or other treatment). Note: A full Manic Episode emerging during antidepressant treatment (medication, electroconvulsive therapy, etc.) but persisting beyond the physiological effect of that treatment is sufficient evidence for a Manic Episode and, therefore, a Bipolar I diagnosis.

(E) <u>Exclude</u> the diagnosis of Bipolar Disorder if during the course of the illness the patient had delusions or hallucinations for at least 2 weeks in the absence of prominent mood symptoms. In such cases the diagnosis is Schizophrenia, Schizoaffective Disorder, Delusional Disorder, Schizophreniform Disorder, or Psychotic Disorder Not Elsewhere Classified.

See pages 28-31 for questions about psychotic symptoms.

Was there a time when you [PSYCHOTIC SX] but did not feel [MANIC MOOD]/have problems with [MANIC SYMPTOMS]?

IF YES:

For how long did you have [PSYCHOTIC SX] only?
When did the [MANIC MOOD/SX] begin in relation to this?

DIAGNOSIS OF BIPOLAR DISORDER

Bipolar I disorder

Requires a history of a manic episode. A history of a depressive episode is not necessary (but usually present).

Bipolar II disorder

Requires a history of a hypomanic episode and a depressive episode. A history of a manic episode rules out the diagnosis of bipolar II disorder, and bipolar I disorder should be diagnosed.

HYPOMANIC EPISODE

Inclusion: A, at least 3 or 4 from B, C, D
Exclusion: E-G

(A) A distinct period of abnormally and persistently elevated, expansive, or irritable mood, and abnormally and persistently increased activity or energy, lasting at least 4 consecutive days and present most of the day nearly every day.

Have there been times lasting at least several days when you felt high, on top of the world, euphoric, or overly cheery?
Have you had periods when you are more energetic or active than usual?

IF YES:

Describe what that was like.
How many periods like this have you had?
Does anything cause this? (Were you using drugs?)
How is this different than a normal good mood?
How long do these periods typically last? (How long was the longest?)
Is your mood/energy/activity elevated almost all day long?

IF NO:

What about a period lasting several days when you were unusually irritable and quick to argue or fight?

IF YES:

Describe what that is like.
Does your energy level seem higher than usual during these times? (Are you more active?)
How many periods like this have you had?
Does anything cause the irritable mood? (Were you using drugs?)
How long do these periods typically last? (How long was the longest?)
During these periods do you feel irritable almost all day?

(Were you hospitalized for any of these periods?)

Now I'm going to ask about some other things that may have occurred at the same time you were feeling [MOOD STATE].

B. During the period of mood disturbance and increased energy or activity, 3 or more of the following symptoms (4 if the mood is only irritable) have persisted, are present to a significant degree, and represent a noticeable change from usual behavior.

(B1) Inflated self-esteem or grandiosity.

What was your self-esteem like during this time?
Did you feel more self-confident than usual?
Did you feel like you had special talents, abilities, or powers?
IF YES: Like what?

When some people feel [HYPOMANIC MOOD] they may think they're going to become famous or do great things. Did you have any thoughts like that? **IF YES:** Like what?

(B2) Decreased need for sleep (e.g., feels rested after only 3 hours of sleep).

During this time how did you sleep?
Did you need less sleep than usual to feel rested?
IF YES: How many hours were you able to get by on?

(B3) More talkative than usual or pressure to keep talking.

Were you more talkative than usual?
Did you talk on and on so that it was hard for others to get a word in?
Did you feel a pressure to talk constantly?
Did you talk faster than you normally do?
IF YES: Did you talk so fast that it was hard to understand you?

(B4) Flight of ideas or subjective experience that thoughts are racing.

During this time did it feel like your thoughts were going very fast or racing through your mind?

(B5) Distractibility (i.e., attention too easily drawn to unimportant or irrelevant external stimuli) as reported or observed.

Were you easily distracted so that any little thing could get you off track? **IF YES:** What was that like?

(B6) Increase in goal-directed activity (either socially, at work or school, or sexually) or psychomotor agitation.

Were you more active than usual? For example, did you do more chores around the house?

Were you so energetic that instead of sleeping you did household chores or work throughout the night?

Did you start new projects or take on added responsibilities?

Did you work more?

Did you call friends more? Were you sexually more active than usual?

Did you feel physically restless so that it was hard to sit still?
Were you always moving or pacing back and forth?

IF YES TO ANY OF ABOVE: Tell me what you did.

(B7) Excessive involvement in activities that have a high potential for painful consequences (e.g., engaging in unrestricted buying sprees, sexual indiscretions, or foolish business investments).

Did you do anything that could have caused problems for you or your family? For example, when some people feel [HYPOMANIC MOOD] they go on spending sprees, write bad checks, invest money foolishly, or do things sexually that are unusual for them. Did you do anything like that?

IF YES: Like what?

(C) The episode is associated with an unequivocal change in functioning that is uncharacteristic of the person when not symptomatic.

What effect did this episode (these episodes) have on your life at the time it was going on?

Were you functioning any better or worse?

Did it cause major problems in your job? School? Marriage? Social life? Relationships with friends or family?

IF YES TO ANY: What happened?

(D) The disturbance in mood and the change in functioning are observable by others.

Did anyone notice that there was something different about you?
IF YES: What did they say?

Did anyone notice that you weren't functioning the way you normally do? **IF YES:** What did they say?

(E) <u>Exclude</u> the diagnosis if the symptoms are severe enough to cause marked impairment in social or occupational functioning, or to necessitate hospitalization. If there are psychotic features the episode is, by definition, manic.

Did you get treatment? (Were you hospitalized?)

Did it cause major problems in your job? School? Marriage? Social life? Relationships with friends or family?
IF YES TO ANY: What happened?

(F) <u>Exclude</u> the diagnosis if the symptoms are attributable to the direct physiological effects of a substance (e.g., a drug of abuse, a medication, or other treatment). Note: A full Hypomanic Episode emerging during antidepressant treatment (medication, electroconvulsive therapy, etc.) but persisting beyond the physiological effect of that treatment is sufficient evidence for a Hypomanic Episode. However, caution is indicated so that one or two symptoms (particularly increased irritability, edginess or agitation following antidepressant use) are not taken as sufficient evidence of a Hypomanic Episode, nor necessarily an indication of a Bipolar Disorder diathesis.

(G) <u>Exclude</u> the diagnosis of Bipolar II Disorder if during the course of the illness the patient had delusions or hallucinations for at least 2 weeks in the absence of prominent mood symptoms. In such cases the diagnosis is Schizophrenia, Schizoaffective Disorder, Delusional Disorder, Schizophreniform Disorder, or Psychotic Disorder Not Elsewhere Classified.

See pages 28-31 for questions about psychotic symptoms.
Was there a time when you [PSYCHOTIC SX] but did not feel [MANIC MOOD]/have problems with [MANIC SYMPTOMS]?
IF YES:
For how long did you have [PSYCHOTIC SX] only?
When did the [MANIC MOOD/SX] begin in relation to this?

MAJOR DEPRESSIVE DISORDER

Inclusion: A1 or A2, at least 5 from A, B
Exclusion: C-E

A. Presence of a Major Depressive Episode. Five (or more) of the following criteria have been present during the same 2-week period and represent a change from previous functioning: at least one of the symptoms is either 1) depressed mood or 2) loss of interest or pleasure.

Note: For each symptom you must inquire about duration (For how long have you...) and persistence (Do you feel like that nearly every day?).

Note: Do not include symptoms that are clearly due to a medical illness.

Note: The normal and expected response to an event involving significant loss (e.g. bereavement, financial ruin, natural disaster, a serious medical illness) may include feelings of intense sadness, rumination about the loss, insomnia, poor appetite and weight loss, which may resemble a depressive episode. Although such symptoms may be understandable and considered appropriate to the loss, the presence of a major depressive episode should be carefully considered. The presence of symptoms such as feelings of worthlessness, suicidal ideas (as distinct from wanting to join a deceased loved one), psychomotor retardation, and severe impairment of overall function suggest the presence of a Major Depressive Episode.

(A1) Depressed mood most of the day, nearly every day, as indicated by either subjective report (e.g., feels sad, empty, or hopeless) or observation made by others (e.g., appears tearful).

How is your mood?
Have you been feeling sad, blue, down, or depressed?
IF YES: For how long have you been feeling that way?
Do you feel that way nearly every day?
How much of the day does it last?

(A2) Markedly diminished interest or pleasure in all, or almost all, activities most of the day, nearly every day as indicated by either subjective account or observation.

Have you lost interest in or get less pleasure from the things you used to enjoy? (Are there things you still enjoy?)
IF YES: How long have you been feeling that way? Is it every day?

(A3) Significant weight loss when not dieting or weight gain (e.g., a change of more than 5% of body weight in a month), or a decrease or increase in appetite nearly every day.

Has there been any change in your appetite?
IF INCREASED OR DECREASED:
How much more/less have you been eating?
Is it like that nearly every day?
For how long has your appetite been increased/decreased?

Have you gained/lost any weight? **IF YES:** How much? Since when?

(A4) Insomnia or hypersomnia nearly every day.

How have you been sleeping?
How many hours per night have you been sleeping? (What time have you been going to sleep? Waking up?)
How does this compare to normal?
IF INCREASED OR DECREASED:
Is it a problem nearly every day?
For how long have you had sleep problems?
IF DECREASED:
Do you have problems falling asleep? (Every night?)
Do you wake up in the middle of the night?
IF YES: How long does it take to get back to sleep?
Do you wake up earlier than you would like?

(A5) Psychomotor agitation or retardation nearly every day (observable by others, not merely subjective feelings of restlessness or being slowed down).

Observation of psychomotor agitation: fidgety while sitting; pacing; pulling on hair, skin, or clothing; handwringing; crossing and uncrossing legs frequently; restless/bouncing legs.
Observation of psychomotor retardation: slowed speech; long pauses before answering questions or between words; mute; slowed body movements.

Agitation: Have you been more fidgety and having problems sitting still? **IF YES:** Have others noticed your restlessness?

Retardation: Have you felt slowed down, like you were moving in slow motion or stuck in mud? **IF YES:** Have others noticed?

(A6) Fatigue or loss of energy nearly every day.

How has your energy level been?

IF UNCERTAIN: I am not talking about lack of interest or motivation, but whether you are feeling tired or worn out?

IF FATIGUED: Duration and persistence questions (top of pg. 40).

(A7) Feelings of worthlessness or excessive or inappropriate guilt (which may be delusional) nearly every day (not merely self-reproach or guilt about being sick).

How has your self-esteem been?

IF LOW: What types of thoughts do you have about yourself?
Do you feel like you're worthless or a failure?

IF YES: Tell me about that.

Have you been blaming yourself for things?
Do you feel guilty?

IF YES: About what?
Do you think about things from the past and feel guilty about them? **IF YES:** Like what?

IF EVIDENCE OF GUILT OR WORTHLESSNESS:

How often do you think [PATIENT'S DESCRIPTION OF GUILT OR WORTHLESSNESS]? (Is it on your mind nearly every day?)

(A8) Diminished ability to think or concentrate, or indecisiveness, nearly every day (either subjective account or as observed by others).

Have you been having problems thinking or concentrating?

IF YES: What does this interfere with?
Are you able to read? Watch TV? Follow a conversation?
Duration and persistence questions

Is it harder to make decisions than is usual for you?

IF YES: What kind of decisions are harder to make?
What about everyday decisions like what to wear, what to eat, etc?
Duration and persistence questions

(A9) Recurrent thoughts of death (not just fear of dying), recurrent suicidal ideation without a specific plan, or a suicide attempt or a specific plan for committing suicide.

Sometimes when a person feels down or depressed they might think about dying. Have you been having any thoughts like that?

Have you thought about taking your life?
IF YES: Tell me about that. (Did you think of a way to do it?) How close have you come to making a suicide attempt?
IF NO: Do you wish you were dead? When you go to sleep, do you often wish you would not wake up?

(B) The symptoms cause clinically significant distress or impairment in social, occupational, or other important areas of functioning.

How much does it bother you that you feel this way?

What difficulties in your life has the depression caused?
Has it affected your job (school)?...marriage?....relationship with friends?.....social life? **IF YES:** In what way?

Does the depression interfere with or keep you from completing your daily routine and chores?

(C) Exclude the diagnosis if the symptoms are attributable to the direct physiological effects of a substance or another medical condition.

(D) Exclude the diagnosis if during the course of the illness the patient had delusions or hallucinations for at least 2 weeks in the absence of prominent mood symptoms. In such cases the diagnosis is Schizophrenia, Schizoaffective Disorder, Delusional Disorder, Schizophreniform Disorder, or Psychotic Disorder Not Elsewhere Classified.

Was there a time when you [PSYCHOTIC SX] but did not feel sad or depressed and have problems with [DEPRESSIVE SX]?
IF YES: For how long did you have [PSYCHOTIC SX] only? When did the depression begin in relation to this?

(E) Exclude the diagnosis if there has been a history of a Manic or Hypomanic Episode.

PERSISTENT DEPRESSIVE DISORDER (DYSTHYMIA)

Inclusion: A, at least 2 from B, C, D, H
Exclusion: E-G

(A) Depressed mood for most of the day, for more days than not, as indicated either by subjective account or observation of others, for at least 2 years.

How is your mood?
Have you been feeling sad, blue, down, or depressed?
IF YES: How often do you feel this way? (On more days than not?)
For how long have you felt this way?
(Has it been at least two years?)

Diagnostic Note: If criteria are met for Major Depressive Disorder for 2 years, then both Major Depression and Persistent Depressive Disorder are diagnosed. However, only Persistent Depressive Disorder should be coded.

(B) Presence, while depressed, of 2 or more of the following:

When you were depressed did you usually...
1)...have a poor appetite or overeat?
2)...have difficulty sleeping or with oversleeping?
3)...feel tired?
4)...feel down on yourself, or have low self-esteem?
5)...have problems concentrating or difficulty making decisions?
6)...feel hopeless or pessimistic about the future?

(C) During the 2-year period of the disturbance, never without the symptoms in Criteria A and B for more than 2 months at a time.

During the past 2 years were you ever free of depression or sadness for a couple of months or more?

Were you ever free of [SYMPTOMS IN B] for a couple of months or more?

(D) Criteria for Major Depressive Disorder may be continuously present for 2 years.

(E) **<u>Exclude</u> the diagnosis if there is a history of a Manic or Hypomanic Episode.**

(F) **<u>Exclude</u> the diagnosis if symptoms are superimposed on a chronic psychotic disorder such as Schizophrenia, Schizoaffective Disorder, Delusional Disorder, or other psychotic disorder.**

(G) **<u>Exclude</u> the diagnosis if the symptoms are due to the direct physiological effects of a substance (e.g., a drug of abuse, a medication), or another medical condition (e.g., hypothyroidism).**

(H) **The symptoms cause clinically significant distress or impairment in social, occupational, or other important areas of functioning.**

How much does it bother you that you feel this way?

What difficulties in your life has the depression caused?
Has it affected your job (school)?....marriage?....relationship with friends?.....social life?
IF YES: In what way?

Does the chronic depression interfere with or keep you from completing your daily routine and chores?

PREMENSTRUAL DYSPHORIC DISORDER

Inclusion: at least 5 from A, B, D
Exclusion: C, E

(A) In the majority of menstrual cycles, the following symptoms must be present in the final week before the onset of menses, start to improve within a few days after the onset of menses, and become minimal or absent in the week post-menses. At least 1 of the symptoms is from the first 4 listed, and the individual must experience 5 or more total symptoms of the 11 listed.

Do you have mood changes in the week before your period?
IF YES: Describe what types of mood changes you have.
How long does it take before the symptoms start to get better?
(By a week after your period are they almost gone?)
Do you experience this before most of your periods?

Let me ask you about specific symptoms that may occur. I am interested in knowing if they occur before most periods, and whether they have resolved, or almost resolved, by a week after your period is over. Do you....

1. have mood swings where you suddenly feel sad or tearful or more sensitive to comments or criticisms of others?
2. feel more irritable or angry or get into more arguments?
3. feel depressed, hopeless, or self-critical?
4. feel anxious, tense, keyed up, or on edge?
5. feel less interested in your usual activities?
6. have problems concentrating?
7. feel very tired?
8. overeat or have food cravings?
9. have difficulty sleeping or sleep too much?
10. feel overwhelmed or out of control emotionally?
11. have breast tenderness or swelling?
    joint or muscle pain?
    feel bloated?
    gain weight?

(B) The symptoms are associated with clinically significant distress or interference with work, school, usual social activities or relationships with others (e.g., avoidance of social activities, decreased productivity and efficiency at work, school or home).

How much does it bother you that you have these symptoms?

What difficulties in your life have the premenstrual symptoms caused? Have they affected your job (school)?....marriage?....relationship with friends?.....social life?

IF YES: In what way?

Do the premenstrual symptoms interfere with or keep you from completing your daily routine and chores?

(C) <u>Exclude</u> the diagnosis if it is merely an exacerbation of the symptoms of another disorder such as Major Depressive Disorder, Panic Disorder, Persistent Depressive Disorder, or a Personality Disorder (although it may co-occur with any of these disorders).

(D) Criterion A should be confirmed by prospective daily ratings during at least two symptomatic cycles. (The diagnosis may be made provisionally prior to this confirmation.)

(E) <u>Exclude</u> the diagnosis if the symptoms are due to the direct physiological effects of a substance (e.g., a drug of abuse, a medication or other treatment), or another medical condition (e.g., hyperthyroidism).

PANIC DISORDER

Inclusion: at least 4 from A, at least 1 from B
Exclusion: C, D

(A) Recurrent unexpected panic attacks. A panic attack is an abrupt surge of intense fear or intense discomfort that reaches a peak within minutes, and during which time 4 or more of the characteristic symptoms occur.

An anxiety or panic attack is a sudden rush of intense fear, anxiety, or discomfort that comes on from out of the blue for no apparent reason, or in situations where you did not expect it to occur. Have you ever experienced this? **IF YES:** During an attack did you...

1. feel your heart racing, pounding, fluttering, or skipping beats?
2. sweat?
3. tremble or shake?
4. have trouble catching your breath, or feel like you were being smothered?
5. feel like you were choking?
6. have chest pain, pressure, tightness, or discomfort?
7. feel nauseated, sick to your stomach, or like you might have diarrhea?
8. feel dizzy, light-headed, unsteady, or like you might faint?
9. have chills or feel hot?
10. feel numbness or tingling in your fingers or feet?
11. feel like things around you were unreal, like you were in a dream, like parts of your body were unreal or detached from you, or like you were outside of yourself, watching?
12. fear you were going crazy or might lose control?
13. fear you might die?

During a bad attack, how long does it usually take from the time it begins until it is at its worst?

IF UNCLEAR OR MORE THAN A FEW MINUTES:

Would the symptoms ever reach their peak quickly, within a few minutes?

How many attacks have you experienced?
Does anything bring them on?

IF SPECIFIC SITUATION DESCRIBED:

Do they only occur in these situations, or do they sometimes come on from out of the blue or in unexpected situations?

(B) At least one of the attacks has been followed by 1 month or more of one or both of the following:
a. Persistent concern or worry about additional panic attacks or their consequences (e.g., losing control, having a heart attack, "going crazy");
b. Significant maladaptive behavior related to the attacks (e.g., behaviors designed to avoid having a panic attack, such as avoidance of exercise or unfamiliar situations).

---

a. Did you worry a lot about having more of them?
IF YES: For how long did you worry about having them?

What were you afraid might happen from these anxiety attacks?
(Did you worry a lot that you might have a heart attack?)
(Did you worry that you might go crazy or lose control?)
IF YES: For how long did you worry about that?

b. Did you change your behavior or routine after the attacks began? (Are there situations or places you avoid to keep from having an attack?)

(C) Exclude the diagnosis if the symptoms are due to the direct physiological effects of a substance (e.g., a drug of abuse, a medication) or another medical condition (e.g., hyperthyroidism, cardiopulmonary disorders).

(D) Exclude the diagnosis if the anxiety is better accounted for by another mental disorder, such as the obsessions in Obsessive-Compulsive Disorder, reminders of traumatic events in Posttraumatic Stress Disorder, separation from attachment figures in Separation Anxiety Disorder, circumscribed phobic objects or situations in Specific Phobia, or feared social situations in Social Anxiety Disorder.

AGORAPHOBIA

Inclusion: A-H
Exclusion: I

Diagnostic Note: In DSM-5-TR agoraphobia is diagnosed as a separate disorder from panic disorder. Patients with panic disorder and agoraphobia should be given 2 diagnoses. Some patients may have agoraphobia without panic disorder.

(A) Marked fear or anxiety of at least 2 of the following situations:

1. **Using public transportation (e.g., automobiles, buses, trains, ships, planes).**
2. **Being in open spaces (e.g., parking lots, marketplaces, bridges).**
3. **Being in enclosed places (e.g., shops, theaters, or cinemas).**
4. **Standing in line or being in a crowd.**
5. **Being outside of the home alone.**

Some people have very strong fears of being in certain places or in certain situations. Do any of the following make you feel very fearful, anxious or nervous?

1. Traveling in a car, bus, boat, train, or plane.
2. Being in open spaces like a parking lot, park, or supermarket.
3. Being on a bridge.
4. Being in movie theaters or stores.
5. Standing in line or being in crowds.
6. Being away from home alone.

(B) The individual fears or avoids these situations because of thoughts that escape might be difficult or help might not be available in the event of developing panic-like symptoms or other incapacitating or embarrassing symptoms (e.g., fear of falling in the elderly, fear of incontinence).

I know it may be difficult to describe, but what is it about [PHOBIC SITUATION] that worries you?
What do you think might happen to you?
What are you afraid of?

(C) The agoraphobic situations almost always provoke fear or anxiety.

How regularly do you get anxious when you [PHOBIC SITUATION]?

(D) The agoraphobic situations are actively avoided, require the presence of a companion, or endured with marked fear or anxiety.

To what degree do you avoid [PHOBIC SITUATION]?
IF NO AVOIDANCE:
So what do you do, how do you cope?
Does having someone with you help?
Do you [PHOBIA] only when you're with someone?
Do you [PHOBIA] alone?
IF YES: How bad does the anxiety get?

(E) The fear or anxiety is out of proportion to the actual danger posed by the agoraphobic situations and to sociocultural context.

(F) The fear, anxiety, or avoidance is persistent, typically lasting six months or more.

For how long have you had the fear of [PHOBIC SITUATION]?

(G) The fear, anxiety, or avoidance causes clinically significant distress or impairment in social, occupational, or other important areas of functioning.

What problems in your life has the avoidance/fear of [PHOBIA] caused?
Has it caused job (or school) problems?
What about marital problems?
What about interfering with friendships?
Has [PHOBIA] affected leisure time activities?
How much does it bother you that you have this fear of [PHOBIA]?

(H) If another medical condition is present (e.g., inflammatory bowel disease, Parkinson's) the fear, anxiety, or avoidance is clearly excessive.

(I) <u>Exclude</u> the diagnosis if the anxiety is better accounted for by another mental disorder, such as the obsessions in Obsessive-Compulsive Disorder, reminders of traumatic events in Posttraumatic Stress Disorder, separation from attachment figures in Separation Anxiety Disorder, circumscribed phobic objects or situations in Specific Phobia, or feared social situations in Social Anxiety Disorder.

SOCIAL ANXIETY DISORDER (SOCIAL PHOBIA)

Inclusion: A-G
Exclusion: H-J

(A) Marked fear or anxiety about one or more social situations in which the individual is exposed to possible scrutiny by others. Examples include social interactions (e.g., having a conversation, meeting unfamiliar people), being observed (e.g., eating or drinking), or performing in front of others (e.g., giving a speech).

Some people feel very anxious in certain social situations in which they might be watched or evaluated by others. Let me ask you about some specific situations. Do any of the following make you feel very fearful, anxious or nervous?

1. Eating in front of others
2. Writing in front of others
3. Public speaking
4. Saying something when in a group of people
5. Asking a question when in a group of people
6. Urinating in public restrooms
7. Business meetings
8. Parties (meeting new people)

IF YES TO ANY: How strong is your anxiety?

(B) The individual fears that he or she will act in a way or show anxiety symptoms that will be negatively evaluated (e.g., be humiliated or embarrassed, or be rejected or offend others).

When [PHOBIA] do you worry a lot that you might do or say something that would embarrass you in front of others, or that other people might think badly of you?

(I know it may be difficult to describe, but what is it about [PHOBIA] that worries you; e.g., embarrassing yourself by choking when eating, hand trembling when writing, being unable to urinate, your mind going blank or losing your train of thought when lecturing or speaking?)

(C) The social situations almost always provoke fear or anxiety.

How regularly do you get anxious when you [PHOBIA]?
(Do you get anxious all of the time, or only some of the time?)

(D) The social situations are actively avoided or endured with intense fear or anxiety.

To what degree do you avoid [PHOBIA]?
IF NO AVOIDANCE:
How bad does the anxiety get when you [PHOBIA]?

(E) The fear or anxiety is out of proportion to the actual threat posed by the social situation and to the sociocultural context.

(F) The fear, anxiety, or avoidance is persistent, typically lasting six months or more.

For how long have you had the fear of [PHOBIA]?

(G) The fear, anxiety, or avoidance causes clinically significant distress or impairment in social, occupational, or other important areas of functioning.

What problems in your life has the avoidance/fear of [PHOBIA] caused?
Has it caused job (or school) problems?
What about marital problems?
What about interfering with friendships?
Has [PHOBIA] affected leisure time activities?
How much does it bother you that you have this fear of [PHOBIA]?

(H) <u>Exclude</u> the diagnosis if the symptoms are due to the direct physiological effects of a substance (e.g., a drug of abuse, a medication) or another medical condition.

(I) <u>Exclude</u> the diagnosis if the anxiety is better accounted for by another mental disorder (e.g., anxiety about having a panic attack in Panic Disorder, agoraphobic situations in Agoraphobia, public exposure to perceived flaws in Body Dysmorphic Disorder).

(J) If another medical condition (e.g., Parkinson's disease, obesity, disfigurement from burn or injury) is present, the fear, anxiety or avoidance is clearly unrelated or is excessive.

SPECIFIC PHOBIA

Inclusion: A-F
Exclusion: G

(A) Marked fear or anxiety about a specific object or situation (e.g., flying, heights, animals, receiving an injection, seeing blood).

Some people have very strong fears of certain objects or situations. Do you have any strong fears of certain objects or situations?
Do any of the following make you feel very fearful or nervous?

1. Heights
2. Cats or dogs
3. Spiders, bugs, snakes, or mice
4. Flying
5. Seeing blood
6. Being in water (e.g., swimming pools, lakes)
7. Storms
8. Receiving an injection

IF YES TO ANY: How strong is your anxiety?

NOTE: Do not include fears related to agoraphobia or social phobia.

(B) The phobic object or situation almost always provokes immediate fear or anxiety.

When you [PHOBIA] how often does it make you feel anxious?
How quickly does the anxiety come on when you [PHOBIA]?

(C) The phobic object or situation is actively avoided, or endured with intense fear or anxiety.

To what degree do you avoid [PHOBIA]?

IF NO AVOIDANCE:

How bad does the anxiety get when you [PHOBIA]?
(How upset do you get when you [PHOBIA]?)

(D) The fear or anxiety is out of proportion to the actual danger posed by the specific object or situation and to the sociocultural context.

(E) The fear, anxiety, or avoidance is persistent, typically lasting six months or more.

For how long have you had the fear of [PHOBIA]?

(F) The fear, anxiety, or avoidance cause clinically significant distress or impairment in social, occupational, or other important areas of functioning.

What problems in your life has the avoidance/fear of [PHOBIA] caused?
Has it caused job (or school) problems?
What about marital problems?
What about interfering with friendships?
Has [PHOBIA] affected leisure time activities?
How much does it bother you that you have this fear of [PHOBIA]?

(G) <u>Exclude</u> the diagnosis if the anxiety is better accounted for by another mental disorder, such as fear and anxiety of situations associated with panic-like symptoms as in Agoraphobia, objects or situation related to obsessions in Obsessive-Compulsive Disorder, reminders of traumatic events in Posttraumatic Stress Disorder, separation from attachment figures in Separation Anxiety Disorder, or feared social situations in Social Anxiety Disorder.

GENERALIZED ANXIETY DISORDER

Inclusion: A, B, at least 3 from C, D
Exclusion: E, F

(A) Excessive anxiety and worry (apprehensive expectation), occurring more days than not for at least 6 months, about a number of events or activities such as work or school performance.

During the past several months, have you frequently been worried or anxious about a number of things in your daily life?

IF YES: What have you worried about?
(Do you worry about your family? Health? Money? School? Work? Other things?)
Do people say that you worry too much?
Do you think you do?
Do you think your anxiety is excessive?
Do you worry that something bad is going to happen to you, or to someone close to you?
How often do you worry about these things? (On more days than not?)
For how long? (Has it been at least six months?)

(B) The individual finds it difficult to control the worry.

Is it hard for you to control or stop your worrying?
IF NO: Then why don't you stop the worrying?

(C) The anxiety and worry are associated with 3 or more of the following six symptoms (with at least some symptoms present for more days than not for the past 6 months).

When you worry do you often…

1. feel restless, fidgety, jittery, keyed up, or on edge?
2. get tired very easily?
3. have problems concentrating, or does your "mind go blank?"
4. feel irritable?
5. feel tension in your muscles?
6. have problems falling asleep or staying asleep? (Or is your sleep restless?)

(D) The anxiety, worry, or physical symptoms cause clinically significant distress or impairment in social, occupational, or other important areas of functioning.

How much does it bother you that you feel this way?
What effect has the anxiety or worry had on your life?
Has it affected your job (school)?....marriage?....relationship with friends?.....social life?.....leisure activities?
IF YES: In what way?

Does the anxiety interfere with or keep you from completing your daily routine and chores?

(E) <u>Exclude</u> the diagnosis if the symptoms are due to the direct physiological effects of a substance (e.g., a drug of abuse, a medication) or another medical condition (e.g., hyperthyroidism).

(F) <u>Exclude</u> the diagnosis if the anxiety is better accounted for by another mental disorder, such as anxiety about panic attacks in Panic Disorder, negative evaluation in Social Anxiety Disorder, contamination or other obsessions in Obsessive-Compulsive Disorder, reminders of traumatic events in Posttraumatic Stress Disorder, separation from attachment figures in Separation Anxiety Disorder, gaining weight in Anorexia Nervosa, physical complaints in Somatic Symptom Disorder, perceived appearance in Body Dysmorphic Disorder, having a serious illness in Illness Anxiety Disorder, or the content of delusional beliefs in Schizophrenia or Delusional Disorder.

POSTTRAUMATIC STRESS DISORDER

Inclusion: at least 1 from A, B, & C; at least 2 from D & E; F,G
Exclusion: H

A. Exposure to actual or threatened death, serious injury, or sexual violence, in 1 or more of the following ways:

(A1) Directly experiencing the traumatic event(s).

Have you ever experienced a traumatic event in which you thought your life was in danger? **IF YES:** What happened?

(What about a traumatic event in which you were, or could have been, seriously injured?) **IF YES:** What happened?

Have you ever been sexually abused? **IF YES:** What happened?

(A2) Witnessing, in person, the traumatic event(s) as they occurred to others.

Have you ever witnessed someone else experience a traumatic event in which their life was in danger? **IF YES:** What happened?

What about witnessing someone getting seriously injured?
IF YES: What happened?

Have you ever seen someone sexually abused?
IF YES: What happened?

(A3) Learning that the traumatic event(s) occurred to a close family member or close friend. In cases of actual or threatened death to a friend or family member the event(s) must have been violent or accidental.

Has a close family member or close friend ever experienced a traumatic event in which they were killed or almost died?
IF YES: What happened?

(A4) Experiencing repeated or extreme exposure to aversive details of the traumatic event(s) (e.g., first responders collecting human remains; police officers repeatedly exposed to details of child abuse). This does not apply to exposure through electronic media, television, movies, or pictures, unless this exposure is work related.

Use information from above questions.

B. Presence of 1 or more of the following intrusion symptoms associated with the traumatic event(s) beginning after the traumatic event(s) occurred:

(B1) Recurrent, involuntary, and intrusive distressing memories of the traumatic event(s).

Do upsetting memories about the [TRAUMA] pop into your head?
IF YES: How frequent are they?

(B2) Recurrent distressing dreams in which the content and/or affect of the dream is related to the traumatic event(s).

Do you have upsetting dreams related to the [TRAUMA]?
IF YES: How frequent are they?

(B3) Dissociative reactions (e.g., flashbacks) in which the individual feels or acts as if the traumatic events(s) are recurring. (Such reactions may occur on a continuum, with the most extreme expression being a complete loss of awareness of present surroundings.)

Some people who [TRAUMA] sometimes have flashbacks where they relive the event, and they may even act or feel as though the event is happening again. Has this happened to you?
IF YES: Describe.

(B4) Intense or prolonged psychological distress at exposure to internal or external cues that symbolize or resemble an aspect of the traumatic event(s).

Are there things that remind you of [TRAUMA] that get you very upset?
IF YES: Describe.

(B5) Marked physiological reactions to internal or external cues that symbolize or resemble an aspect of the traumatic event(s).

Do reminders of [TRAUMA] make you tremble, break out into a sweat, hyperventilate, or have a racing heart?
IF YES: Describe.

C. Persistent avoidance of stimuli associated with the traumatic event(s), beginning after the traumatic event(s) occurred, as evidenced by 1 or more of the following:

(C1) Avoidance of, or efforts to avoid, distressing memories, thoughts, or feelings about or closely associated with the traumatic event(s).

Do you try to block out thoughts or feelings related to [TRAUMA]?

(C2) Avoidance of, or efforts to avoid, external reminders (people, places, conversations, activities, objects, situations) that arouse distressing memories, thoughts or feelings about, or that are closely associated with, the traumatic event(s).

Do you try to avoid activities, situations, or places that remind you of the [TRAUMA]? **IF YES:** Like what?
Do you avoid people who remind you of it?
Do you avoid talking about it?

D. Negative alterations in cognitions and mood associated with the traumatic event(s), beginning or worsening after the traumatic event(s) occurred, as evidenced by 2 or more of the following:

(D1) Inability to remember an important aspect of the traumatic event(s) (typically due to dissociative amnesia and not due to other factors such as head injury, alcohol, or drugs).

Are there some aspects of the [TRAUMA] that you can't recall?
IF YES: Like what?

(D2) Persistent and exaggerated negative beliefs or expectations about oneself, others, or the world (e.g., "I am bad," "No one can be trusted," "The world is completely dangerous" or "My whole nervous system is permanently ruined").

Some people who [TRAUMA] have a very negative view of others, themselves, or the world. Would you say that is true of you?
IF YES: Describe.

Do you believe that you are a bad person?
Do you believe that the world is a completely dangerous place, or that no one can be trusted?
IF YES TO EITHER: Tell me more about that.

(D3) Persistent, distorted cognitions about the cause or consequences of the traumatic event(s) that lead the individual to blame him/herself or others.

Do you blame yourself for [TRAUMA] or its consequences? (What do you think you should have done differently?)

Who else do you blame for what happened? (Tell me about it.)

(D4) Persistent negative emotional state (e.g., fear, horror, anger, guilt, or shame).

Over the past few years have you been chronically and persistently.....
...fearful?...angry?...guilty?...felt ashamed?

(D5) Markedly diminished interest or participation in significant activities.

Have you noticed that since [TRAUMA] you've lost interest in some things you used to enjoy? **IF YES:** Like what?

Are there any activities that you no longer participate in since it occurred? **IF YES:** Like what?

(D6) Feelings of detachment or estrangement from others.

Do you frequently feel like you don't fit in with the people around you? That is, you're with them physically, but you feel distant and cutoff from them.

(D7) Persistent inability to experience positive emotions (e.g., inability to experience happiness, satisfaction, or loving feelings).

Does it seem like you've lost the ability to feel certain positive emotions? **IF YES:** Like what?

Do you feel emotionally numb?

(Has it seemed like you do not experience strong positive feelings about anything, or that you can't feel love anymore?)

E. Marked alterations in arousal and reactivity associated with the traumatic event(s), beginning or worsening after the traumatic event(s) occurred, as evidenced by 2 or more of the following:

(E1) Irritable behavior and angry outbursts (with little or no provocation) typically expressed as verbal or physical aggression toward people or objects.

Do you get easily irritated or lose your temper easily?
Have you had angry outbursts?
IF YES TO EITHER: Describe what that has been like?

(E2) Reckless or self-destructive behavior.

Would you say that you engaged in a pattern of reckless or self-destructive behavior? **IF YES:** Describe.

(E3) Hypervigilance.

Since [TRAUMA] have you been hyperalert, always keeping your guard up with an eye out for possible trouble?

(E4) Exaggerated startle response.

Are you jumpy and easily startled?
IF YES: Describe.

(E5) Problems with concentration.

Since [TRAUMA] have you had problems concentrating?
IF YES: In what areas?

(E6) Sleep disturbance (e.g., difficulty falling or staying asleep or restless sleep).

Since [TRAUMA] have you had problems sleeping?
IF YES: What type of problems?

(F) Duration of the disturbance (Criteria B,C,D, and E) is more than 1 month.

For how long have you been bothered by [SYMPTOMS IN B-E]?

(G) The disturbance causes clinically significant distress or impairment in social, occupational, or other important areas of functioning.

What effect has [TRAUMA] had on your life?
Has it affected your job (school)?....marriage?....relationship with friends?.....social life?.....leisure activities?
IF YES: In what way?

Do the symptoms interfere with or keep you from completing your daily routine and chores?

How much do the [TRAUMA SYMPTOMS] bother you?

(H) <u>Exclude</u> the diagnosis if the symptoms are due to the direct physiological effects of a substance (e.g., medication, drugs, or alcohol) or another medical condition (e.g., traumatic brain injury).

ACUTE STRESS DISORDER

Inclusion: at least 1 from A; at least 9 from B; C, D
Exclusion: E

A. Exposure to actual or threatened death, serious injury, or sexual violation, in 1 or more of the following ways:

(A1) Directly experiencing the traumatic event(s).

Have you ever experienced a traumatic event in which you thought your life was in danger? **IF YES:** What happened?

(What about a traumatic event in which you were, or could have been, seriously injured?) **IF YES:** What happened?

Have you ever been sexually abused? **IF YES:** What happened?

(A2) Witnessing, in person, the event(s) as it occurred to others.

Have you ever witnessed someone else experience a traumatic event in which their life was in danger? **IF YES:** What happened?

What about witnessing someone getting seriously injured?
IF YES: What happened?

Have you ever seen someone sexually abused?
IF YES: What happened?

(A3) Learning that the traumatic event(s) occurred to a close family member or close friend. In cases of actual or threatened death of a family member or friend the event(s) must have been violent or accidental.

Has a close family member or close friend ever experienced a traumatic event in which they were seriously hurt, assaulted or killed?
IF YES: What happened?

(A4) Experiencing repeated or extreme exposure to aversive details of the traumatic event(s) (e.g., first responders collecting human remains; police officers repeatedly exposed to details of child abuse). This does not apply to exposure through electronic media, television, movies, or pictures, unless this exposure is work related.

Use information from above questions.

B. Presence of 9 or more of the following symptoms after the traumatic event(s) occurred:

INTRUSION SYMPTOMS

(B1) Recurrent, involuntary, and intrusive distressing memories of the traumatic event(s).

Do upsetting memories about the [TRAUMA] pop into your head?
IF YES: How frequent are they?

(B2) Recurrent distressing dreams in which the content and/or affect of the dream is related to the event(s).

Do you have upsetting dreams related to the [TRAUMA]?
IF YES: How frequent are they?

(B3) Dissociative reactions (e.g., flashbacks) in which the individual feels or acts as if the traumatic events(s) are recurring. (Such reactions may occur on a continuum, with the most extreme expression being a complete loss of awareness of present surroundings.)

Some people who [TRAUMA] sometimes have flashbacks where they relive the event, and they may even act or feel as though the event is happening again. Has this happened to you? **IF YES:** Describe.

(B4) Intense or prolonged psychological distress or marked physiological reactions in response to internal or external cues that symbolize or resemble an aspect of the traumatic event(s).

Are there things that remind you of [TRAUMA] that get you upset?
IF YES: Describe.

Do reminders of [TRAUMA] make you tremble, break out into a sweat, hyperventilate, or have a racing heart? **IF YES:** Describe.

NEGATIVE MOOD

(B5) Persistent inability to experience positive emotions (e.g., inability to experience happiness, satisfaction, or loving feelings).

Does it seem like you've lost the ability to feel certain positive emotions? **IF YES:** Like what?

Do you feel emotionally numb?
(Has it seemed like you do not experience strong positive feelings about anything, or that you can't feel love anymore?)

DISSOCIATIVE SYMPTOMS

(B6) An altered sense of the reality of one's surroundings or oneself (e.g., seeing oneself from another's perspective, being in a daze, time slowing).

Have you felt like you are "in a daze?"

Are you are less aware of everything going on around you?

At times, does it seem like things are unreal, or like everything was a dream?

(B7) Inability to remember an important aspect of the traumatic event(s) (typically due to dissociative amnesia and not to other factors such as head injury, alcohol, or drugs).

Are there holes in your memory related to the [TRAUMA]?
Are there some aspects of the [TRAUMA] that you can't recall?
IF YES: Like what?

AVOIDANCE SYMPTOMS

(B8) Efforts to avoid distressing memories, thoughts, or feelings about or closely associated with the traumatic event(s).

Do you try to block out thoughts or feelings related to [TRAUMA]?

(B9) Efforts to avoid external reminders (people, places, conversations, activities, objects, situations) that arouse distressing memories, thoughts or feelings about, or that are closely associated with, the traumatic event(s).

Do you try to avoid activities, situations, or places that remind you of [TRAUMA]? **IF YES:** Like what?
Do you avoid people who remind you of it?
Do you avoid talking about it?

AROUSAL SYMPTOMS

(B10) Sleep disturbance (e.g., difficulty falling or staying asleep or restless sleep).

Since [TRAUMA] have you had problems sleeping?
IF YES: What type of problems?

(B11) Irritable behavior and angry outbursts (with little or no provocation) typically expressed as verbal or physical aggression toward people or objects.

Have you been irritable or lost your temper easily?
Have you had angry outbursts?
IF YES TO EITHER: Describe what that has been like.

(B12) Hypervigilance.

Since [TRAUMA] have you been hyperalert, always keeping your guard up with an eye out for possible trouble?

(B13) Problems with concentration.

Since [TRAUMA] have you had problems concentrating?
IF YES: In what areas?

(B14) Exaggerated startle response.

Are you jumpy and easily startled?
IF YES: Describe.

(C) Duration of the disturbance (symptoms in Criterion B) is 3 days to 1 month after trauma exposure.

For how long have you been bothered by [SYMPTOMS IN B]?

(D) The disturbance causes clinically significant distress or impairment in social, occupational, or other important areas of functioning.

What effect has [TRAUMA] had on your life?
Has it affected your job (school)?....marriage?....relationship with friends?.....social life?.....leisure activities?
IF YES: In what way?

Do the symptoms interfere with or keep you from completing your daily routine and chores?

(E) <u>Exclude</u> the diagnosis if the symptoms are due to the direct physiological effects of a substance (e.g., medication, drugs, or alcohol) or another medical condition (e.g., traumatic brain injury) and is not better explained by Brief Psychotic Disorder.

PROLONGED GRIEF DISORDER

Inclusion: A, at least 1 from B, at least 3 from C, D, E
Exclusion: F

A. Death of a person who was close to the bereaved at least 1 year ago

Has anyone close to you passed away?
IF YES: Who was it? When did they pass away?
How has it affected you?

B. Since the death, presence of 1 or more of the following symptoms on most days and nearly every day for at least the past month:

(B1) Intense yearning or longing for the deceased person.

How much do you miss your [DECEASED]?
Do you find yourself still wishing that your [DECEASED] was still here?
In what ways do you still hold onto your [DECEASED]?
How much do you still yearn or long for [DECEASED]?
IF YES TO ANY: Has it felt that way almost every day of the past month?

(B2) Preoccupation with thoughts or memories of the deceased person.

How much do you think about [DECEASED]?
Has it felt that way almost every day of the past month?

C. Since the death 3 or more of the following symptoms have been present to a clinically significant degree, and the symptoms were present nearly every day for at least the past month.

(C1) Identity disruption (e.g., feeling as though a part of oneself has died) since the death

Since [DECEASED] died, have you felt you lost a part of yourself? Like a part of you also died?
IF YES: Can you describe what that is like?
Has it felt that way almost every day of the past month?
How has this feeling affected your functioning?
How has it affected relationships?

(C2) Marked sense of disbelief about the death.

Was it hard to believe that [DECEASED] died?
IF YES: Is it still hard to believe?
Has it felt that way almost every day in the past month?

(C3) Avoidance of reminders that the person is dead.

Do you try to avoid activities, situations, or places that remind you of [DECEASED] or that [DECEASED] is gone?
Do you avoid people who remind you of [DECEASED]?
IF YES: How often have you avoided in the past month?

(C4) Intense emotional pain (e.g., anger, bitterness, sorrow) related to the death.

How much pain have you been in because of his/her death?
Do you feel bitter about the loss?
IF YES: How often have you felt this way in the past month?

(C5) Difficulty reintegrating into one's relationships and activities after the death (e.g., problems engaging with friends, pursuing interests, or planning for the future).

To what degree have you not gotten back to your life since [DECEASED] passed away?
(Are you socializing like usual?)
(Participating in the activities you used to do?)
(Thinking about the future like you used to?)
(Anything else that you no longer do like you used to?)

(C6) Emotional numbness (absence or marked reduction of emotional experience) as a result of the death.

Have you felt emotionally numb since [DECEASED] passed away?
IF YES: How often have you felt this way in the past month?

(C7) Feeling that life is meaningless as a result of the death.

Has life seemed meaningless since [DECEASED] passed away?
IF YES: How often have you felt this way in the past month?

(C8) Intense loneliness as a result of the death.

Since [DECEASED] passed away have you been feeling lonely?
IF YES: How bad has the feeling of loneliness been?
How often have you felt this way in the past month?

D. The disturbance causes clinically significant distress or impairment in social, occupational, or other important areas of functioning.

IF NOT ALREADY KNOWN

What effect has [DECEASED]'s death had on your life?
Has it affected your job? (school?)....marriage?....relationship with friends?.....social life?.....leisure activities?
IF YES: In what way?

Has it interfered with or keep you from completing your daily routine and chores?

E. The duration and severity of the bereavement reaction clearly exceed expected social, cultural, or religious norms for the individual's culture and context.

F. <u>Exclude</u> the diagnosis if the symptoms are better explained by another mental disorder, such as major depressive disorder or posttraumatic stress disorder, and are not attributable to the physiological effects of a substance (e.g., medication, alcohol) or another medical condition.

ADJUSTMENT DISORDER

Inclusion: A, at least 1 from B
Exclusion: C, D, E

(A) The development of emotional or behavioral symptoms in response to an identifiable stressor occurring within 3 months of the onset of the stressor.

Did anything happen before your [SYMPTOMS] began?

B. The symptoms or behaviors are clinically significant, as evidenced by 1 or both of the following:

(B1) Marked distress that is out of proportion to the severity or intensity of the stressor, taking into account the external context and cultural factors that might influence symptom severity and presentation

How much do your {SYMPTOMS] upset you?

(B2) Significant impairment in social, occupational, or other important areas of functioning.

What effect have [SYMPTOMS] had on your life?
Has it affected your job (schooll?)....marriage?....relationship with friends?.....social life?.....leisure activities?
IF YES: In what way?

(C) <u>Exclude</u> the diagnosis if the symptoms meet the criteria for another mental disorder and is not merely an exacerbation of a preexisting mental disorder.

(D) <u>Exclude</u> the diagnosis if the symptoms represent normal bereavement or are explained by prolonged grief disorder.

(E) <u>Exclude</u> the diagnosis if the symptoms last more than 6 months after the stressor or its consequences have terminated.

OBSESSIVE-COMPULSIVE DISORDER

Inclusion: A1 & A2 for obsessions and/or compulsions, B
Exclusion: C, D

(A) Presence of obsessions, compulsions, or both.
<u>Obsessions</u> require <u>both</u> of the following:

1. **Recurrent and persistent thoughts, urges, or images that are experienced, at some time during the disturbance, as intrusive and unwanted and that in most individuals cause marked anxiety or distress.**
2. **The individual attempts to ignore or suppress such thoughts, urges, or images, or to neutralize them with some other thought or action (i.e., by performing a compulsion).**

<u>Compulsions</u> require <u>both</u> of the following:

1. **Repetitive behaviors (e.g., hand washing, ordering, checking) or mental acts (e.g., praying, counting, repeating words silently) that the individual feels driven to perform in response to an obsession, or according to rules that must be applied rigidly.**
2. **The behaviors or mental acts are aimed at preventing or reducing anxiety or distress, or preventing some dreaded event or situation; however, these behaviors or mental acts are not connected in a realistic way with what they are designed to neutralize or prevent, or are clearly excessive.**

<u>Obsessions</u>

1. Some people are bothered by recurrent thoughts or urges or images that seem inappropriate or do not make sense, but they keep repeating over and over and are difficult to get out of their mind. (For example, intrusive, repeated thoughts that you might hurt or kill someone you love even though you don't want to; that the house is unlocked and will be robbed; that the iron or stove is not turned off and the house will burn down; that you will yell obscenities in public; that you are contaminated by germs or dirt; that you hit someone while driving). Has anything like this been a problem for you?

   IF YES: Describe what it's like.
   How often does it happen?
   How do you feel when you have these thoughts?

2. What do you do in response to these thoughts (images)?
   (Do you try to ignore them or put them out of your mind?)
   Do you say things to yourself (or imagine certain other images) in order to counteract the intrusive thought/image?

<u>Compulsions</u>

1. Some people are bothered by having to do something over and over that they can't resist when they try. For example, they wash their hands repeatedly, clean their countertops excessively, repeatedly check whether the door is locked or the stove is turned off, or count things excessively. Have you had any difficulties like this?

   IF YES: Describe what it's like.

   Do you have any rituals that you always have had to do in a particular order, and if the order is wrong you have to start over from the beginning? **IF YES:** Like what?

2. If you do not [COMPULSION], do you get very anxious or tense?

   IF NO: So, why do you do it?

   What do you think might happen if you didn't [COMPULSION]?

(B) The obsessions or compulsions are time consuming (e.g., take more than 1 hour a day) or cause clinically significant distress or impairment in social, occupational, or other important areas of functioning.

How much does it bother you that you have the (OBSESSIONS/ COMPULSIONS)?

What effect has it had on your life?

Has it affected your job (school)?....marriage?....relationship with friends?.....social life?.....leisure activities?

IF YES: In what way?

Does it keep you from completing your daily routine and chores?

How much time a day do you spend (OBSESSION/COMPULSION)?

(C) <u>Exclude</u> the diagnosis if the symptoms are due to the direct physiological effects of a substance (e.g., a drug of abuse, a medication) or another medical condition.

(D) <u>Exclude</u> the diagnosis if the obsessions/compulsions are better accounted for by another mental disorder, such as excessive worries in Generalized Anxiety Disorder, ritualized eating behavior in Eating Disorder, hair pulling in Trichotillomania, skin picking in Excoriation Disorder, difficulty getting rid of possessions in Hoarding Disorder, preoccupation with appearance in Body Dysmorphic Disorder, preoccupation with illness in Illness Anxiety Disorder.

HOARDING DISORDER

Inclusion: A-D
Exclusion: E, F

(A) Persistent difficulty discarding or parting with possessions, regardless of their actual value.

Some people find it very difficult to throw things away. Does that sound like you?

IF YES: What kinds of things do you keep?

IF NO: Have others complained or teased you about how much stuff you save?

IF YES: What did they say?

(B) The difficulty is due to a perceived need to save the items and distress associated with discarding them.

Why do you keep [ACCUMULATED ITEMS]?
How do you feel when you throw out or think about throwing out [ACCUMULATED ITEMS]?

(C) The difficulty discarding possessions results in the accumulation of possessions that congest and clutter active living areas and substantially compromises their intended use. If living areas are uncluttered, it is only because of the interventions of third parties (e.g., family members, cleaners, authorities).

How cluttered is your home because of [ACCUMULATED ITEMS]?
(Which rooms are the worst?)
(Are you unable to use some rooms because there is so much stuff in them?)

IF NO CLUTTER: Has anyone cleaned up your stuff to keep the clutter manageable? **IF YES:** Describe.

(D) The hoarding causes clinically significant distress or impairment in social, occupational, or other important areas of functioning (including maintaining a safe environment for self and others).

How much does it bother you that you have difficulty throwing out [ACCUMULATED ITEMS]?
What effect has saving [ACCUMULATED ITEMS] had on your life?
Has it affected your job (school)?....marriage?....relationship with friends?.....social life?.....leisure activities?
IF YES: In what way?

Has anyone ever said that it is not safe to be in your house/apartment?

(E) <u>Exclude</u> the diagnosis if the symptoms are due to another medical condition (e.g., brain injury, cerebrovascular disease, Prader-Willi syndrome).

(F) <u>Exclude</u> the diagnosis if the hoarding is better accounted for by another mental disorder, such as obsessions in Obsessive-Compulsive Disorder, decreased energy in Major Depressive Disorder, delusions in Schizophrenia or another Psychotic Disorder, cognitive deficits in Dementia, restricted interests in Autism Spectrum Disorder.

BODY DYSMORPHIC DISORDER

Inclusion: A-C
Exclusion: D

(A) Preoccupation with one or more perceived defects or flaws in physical appearance that are not observable or appear slight to others.

Do you often think there is something wrong with the way you look?
Do you often think you look gross, disfigured, or ugly?

IF YES TO EITHER:

To what are you referring?
How much do you think about this?
How hard is it to get your mind off of this?
Have you talked to your friends or family about this?

IF YES:

What do they say?
Do they try to convince you that you are wrong and that you don't look the way you think you do?

(B) At some point during the course of the disorder the person has performed repetitive behaviors (e.g., mirror checking, excessive grooming, skin picking, or reassurance seeking) or mental acts (e.g., comparing their appearance with that of others) in response to the appearance concerns.

Because of your concerns about your appearance are there things that you do over and over?

IF YES: Like what?

Because of your concerns about your appearance how often do you....

...check how you look in the mirror?
...check how you look in other reflective surfaces?
...pick your skin to make it look better?
...ask others if you look okay?
...compare your appearance to others?

(C) The preoccupation causes clinically significant distress or impairment in social, occupational, or other important areas of functioning.

How much does it bother you that you think so much about how you look?

What effect has your preoccupation with how your [BODY PART] looks had on your life?

Has it affected your job (school)?....marriage?....relationship with friends?.....social life?.....leisure activities?
IF YES: In what way?

(D) <u>Exclude</u> the diagnosis if the appearance preoccupations are better accounted for by concerns with body fat or weight in an Eating Disorder.

EXCORIATION (SKIN PICKING) DISORDER

Inclusion: A-C
Exclusion: D, E

(A) Recurrent skin picking resulting in skin lesions.

Do you frequently pick your skin?
IF YES: Where on your body do you pick your skin?
Can you see marks on your skin where you pick?

(B) Repeated attempts to decrease or stop skin picking.

How often have you tried to cut down or stop picking?

(C) The skin picking causes clinically significant distress or impairment in social, occupational, or other important areas of functioning.

How much does it bother you that you pick your skin?
What effect has this had on your life?
Has it affected your job (school)?....marriage?....relationship with friends?.....social life?.....leisure activities?
IF YES: In what way?

(D) <u>Exclude</u> the diagnosis if the skin picking is due to the direct physiological effects of a substance (e.g., cocaine) or another medical condition (e.g., scabies).

(E) <u>Exclude</u> the diagnosis if the skin picking is better accounted for by another mental disorder (e.g., delusions or tactile hallucinations in a Psychotic Disorder, to improve a perceived defect or flaw in appearance in Body Dysmorphic Disorder, stereotypes in Stereotypic Movement Disorder, or intent to harm oneself in Nonsuicidal self-injury).

TRICHOTILLOMANIA (HAIR PULLING DISORDER)

Inclusion: A-C
Exclusion: D, E

(B) Recurrent pulling out of one's hair resulting in hair loss.

Do you frequently pull out your hair from your head, eyebrows, or other parts of your body?

IF YES: Where on your body do you pull your hair?

(B) Repeated attempts to decrease or stop hair pulling.

How often have you tried to cut down or stop pulling out your hair from [BODY AREA]?

(C) The hair pulling causes clinically significant distress or impairment in social, occupational, or other important areas of functioning.

How much does it bother you that you pull out your hair?
What effect has this had on your life?
Has it affected your job (school)?....marriage?....relationship with friends?.....social life?.....leisure activities?

IF YES: In what way?

(D) <u>Exclude</u> the diagnosis if the hair pulling is attributable to another medical condition (e.g., a dermatological condition).

(E) <u>Exclude</u> the diagnosis if the hair pulling is better accounted for by another mental disorder (e.g., hair pulling to improve a perceived defect or flaw in appearance in Body Dysmorphic Disorder).

INTERMITTENT EXPLOSIVE DISORDER

Inclusion: at least 1 from A, B-E
Exclusion: F

(A) Recurrent behavioral outbursts representing a failure to control aggressive impulses as manifest by <u>either</u>:

A1. Verbal aggression (e.g., temper tantrums, tirades, verbal arguments or fights) or physical aggression toward property, animals, or other individuals, occurring twice weekly, on average, for a period of 3 months. The physical aggression does not result in damage or destruction of property and does not result in physical injury to animals or other individuals.

A2. Three behavioral outbursts involving damage or destruction of property and/or physical assault involving physical injury against animals or other individuals occurring within a 12-month period.

A1. Now I'd like to ask you some questions about your temper and violent behavior. Do you have an explosive or violent temper? Do you have verbal temper outbursts? Do you break objects? Have you hit animals in anger?

IF NO: Would others say you have a bad temper?

IF EVIDENCE OF AGGRESSION:

How often do you lose your temper physically/verbally?

A2. Have you ever "lost control" and either hit someone or destroyed property?

IF YES: Describe what happened.
How often has this happened in the past year?

IF UNCLEAR: Have you ever assaulted anyone?
Destroyed property?
How often has this happened in the past year?

(B) The magnitude of aggressiveness expressed during the recurrent outbursts is grossly out of proportion to the provocation or any precipitating psychosocial stressors.

What usually leads up to these temper outbursts?

Do you think your reaction was unreasonable or excessive?

IF NO: Tell me about that.

(C) The recurrent aggressive outbursts are not premeditated (i.e., they are impulsive) and are not committed to achieve some tangible objective (e.g., money, power, intimidation, etc.).

Are your temper outbursts typically planned?
What are you trying to gain from losing your temper?

(D) The recurrent aggressive outbursts cause either marked distress in the individual, or impairment in occupational or interpersonal functioning, or are associated with financial or legal consequences.

How much do the temper/aggressive outbursts bother you?
What effect has this had on your life?
Has it affected your job (school)?....marriage?....relationship with friends?.....social life?
IF YES: In what way?
Have there been any legal issues related to your temper?
How much has your temper cost you financially?

(E) Chronological age is at least 6 years (or equivalent developmental level).

(F) <u>Exclude</u> the diagnosis if the aggressive outbursts are better accounted for by another mental disorder (e.g., Major Depressive Disorder, Bipolar Disorder, Disruptive Mood Dysregulation Disorder, a Psychotic Disorder, Antisocial Personality Disorder, Borderline Personality Disorder), a general medical condition (e.g., head trauma, Alzheimer's Disorder), or due to the direct physiological effects of a substance (e.g., a drug of abuse or medication).

ILLNESS ANXIETY DISORDER

Inclusion: A-E
Exclusion: F

(A) Preoccupation with having or acquiring a serious illness.

Do you often think about the possibility that you have, or will get, some type of serious illness?
IF YES: What do you think you have (will get)?
What makes you worry about this?
How hard is it to get your mind off of this?

(B) Somatic symptoms are not present or, if present, are only mild in intensity. If another medical condition is present or there is a high risk for developing a medical condition (e.g., strong family history is present), the preoccupation is clearly excessive or disproportionate.

Have you been experiencing any physical pain or medical symptoms?
IF YES: What physical symptoms do you have?
Does [SOMATIC SYMPTOMS] bother you a lot?
How much do [SOMATIC SYMPTOMS] disrupt your life?

Note: The presence of significantly bothersome or disruptive somatic symptoms <u>excludes</u> the diagnosis of illness anxiety disorder.

(C) There is a high level of anxiety about health, and the individual is easily alarmed about personal health status.

How anxious do you get when you hear someone is sick?

How anxious are you about your health?

Do you get very anxious about your health pretty easily?

(D) The individual performs excessive health-related behaviors (e.g., repeatedly checks his or her body for signs of illness), or exhibits maladaptive avoidance (e.g., avoiding doctor appointments and hospitals).

How often do you check your body for signs of illness?

How often do you look up health-related information on the internet?

How much time do you spend going to the doctor? (Do you avoid doctor's appointments?)

(E) Illness preoccupation has been present for at least 6 months, but the specific illness that is feared may change over that period of time.

For how long have you been worrying about having or getting a serious illness?

(F) Exclude the diagnosis if the illness-related preoccupation is better accounted for by another mental disorder, such as Somatic Symptom Disorder, Panic Disorder, Generalized Anxiety Disorder, Body Dysmorphic Disorder, Obsessive Compulsive Disorder, or Delusional Disorder, Somatic Type.

SOMATIC SYMPTOM DISORDER

Inclusion: A-C
Exclusion: none

(A) One or more somatic symptoms that are distressing and/or result in significant disruption in daily life.

Have you been experiencing any physical pain or medical symptoms?
IF YES: What physical symptoms do you have?
Does [SOMATIC SYMPTOMS] bother you a lot?
How much do [SOMATIC SYMPTOMS] disrupt your life?

B. Excessive thoughts, feelings, and behaviors related to these somatic symptoms or associated health concerns. At least 1 of the following 3 criteria must be present:

(B1) Disproportionate and persistent thoughts about the seriousness of one's symptoms.

Do you think a lot about the [SOMATIC SYMPTOMS]?
IF YES: What do you think might be wrong?
How hard is it to get your mind off of this?
For how long have you been concerned about this?

(B2) Persistently high level of anxiety about health or symptoms.

How anxious are you about your health? (For how long have you felt this anxious about your health?)

How much do you worry about [SOMATIC SYMPTOMS]? (For how long have you worried about [SOMATIC SYMPTOMS]?

(B3) Excessive time and energy devoted to these symptoms or health concerns.

What effect has your worrying about your health had on your life?
How much time do you spend going to the doctor?
How much time do you spend on the internet looking into this?

(C) Although any one symptom may not be continuously present, the state of being symptomatic is persistent (typically > 6 months).

ATTENTION DEFICIT/HYPERACTIVITY DISORDER—Adult

Inclusion: At least 5 from A1 or A2, B, C, D
Exclusion: E

A. EITHER A1 OR A2:

A1. Inattention: Five (or more) of the following symptoms have persisted for at least 6 months to a degree that is inconsistent with developmental level and that negatively impacts directly on social and academic/occupational activities.

Note: The interview questions in this section are written from the perspective of interviewing an adult. Questions for assessing children are on pages 98-103. The criteria are the same for adults and children.

1. Often fails to give close attention to details or makes careless mistakes in schoolwork, at work, or during other activities (e.g., overlooks or misses details, work is inaccurate).

Do you often make careless mistakes at work, school, or at home?
How often do you have difficulty paying close attention to details?
IF YES TO EITHER: Examples.
Is that the way you normally are?
Have you been this way most of your life?

IF EVIDENCE OF SYMPTOM: Were you like this as a child also? (Beginning at what age?)

2. Often has difficulty sustaining attention in tasks or play activities (e.g., has difficulty remaining focused during lectures, conversations, or lengthy reading).

Some people have a hard time staying on track or paying attention to what they are doing. How often is it difficult for you to concentrate on one thing for a long time?
Is it hard to focus on a task for a long time?
IF YES TO EITHER: Examples.
Is that the way you normally are?
Have you been this way most of your life?

IF EVIDENCE OF SYMPTOM: Were you like this as a child also? (Beginning at what age?)

3. Often does not seem to listen when spoken to directly (e.g., mind seems elsewhere even in the absence of obvious distraction).

How often do you have problems focusing on what others say to you, even when they are speaking directly to you?
Have others commented that you don't seem to be listening?

IF YES TO EITHER: Is that the way you normally are?
Have you been this way most of your life?

IF EVIDENCE OF SYMPTOM: Were you like this as a child also? (Beginning at what age?)

4. Often does not follow through on instructions and fails to finish schoolwork, chores, or duties in the workplace (e.g., starts tasks but quickly loses focus and is easily sidetracked).

Some people have difficulty completing tasks. They start one thing and move on to another before completing the first one. Does that sound like you? (Are there things you don't get done?)

IF YES: Is that the way you normally are?
Have you been this way most of your life?

IF EVIDENCE OF SYMPTOM: Were you like this as a child also? (Beginning at what age?)

5. Often has difficulty organizing tasks and activities (e.g., difficulty managing sequential tasks; difficulty keeping materials and belongings in order; messy, disorganized work; poor time management; tends to fail to meet deadlines).

Is being organized difficult for you? **IF YES:** Tell me about that.
Is it difficult for you to plan and organize your work or household chores?
Is your work space, or home, messy and disorganized?

Are you poor in managing your time? **IF YES:** Examples.
Do you tend to miss deadlines? **IF YES:** Examples.

IF YES TO ANY: Is that the way you normally are?
Have you been this way most of your life?

IF EVIDENCE OF SYMPTOM: Were you like this as a child also? (Beginning at what age?)

6. Often avoids, dislikes, or is reluctant to engage in tasks that require sustained mental effort (e.g., schoolwork or homework, preparing reports, completing forms, or reviewing lengthy papers).

Some people strongly dislike doing things that require a lot of concentration. Are you like that?
Do you often avoid or put off doing a task that requires a lot of concentration? Examples.

IF YES TO EITHER: Is that the way you normally are?
Have you been this way most of your life?

IF EVIDENCE OF SYMPTOM: Were you like this as a child also? (Beginning at what age?)

7. Often loses things necessary for tasks or activities (e.g., school materials, pencils, books, tools, wallets, keys, paperwork, eyeglasses, or mobile telephones).

Do you think that you misplace or lose things like your wallet, keys, cell phone, books, etc. more than most other people do?

IF YES: Like what? How often?
Is that the way you normally are?
Have you been this way most of your life?

IF EVIDENCE OF SYMPTOM: Were you like this as a child also? (Beginning at what age?)

8. Is often easily distracted by extraneous stimuli (may include unrelated thoughts).

Is it difficult for you to keep your mind on the things you want to do because you are easily distracted?

IF YES: What kinds of things distract you?
How common is this?
Does it happen at work? At home?
Is this the way you normally are?
Have you been this way most of your life?

IF EVIDENCE OF SYMPTOM: Were you like this as a child also? (Beginning at what age?)

9. Is often forgetful in daily activities (e.g., doing chores, running errands, returning calls, paying bills, keeping appointments).

Are you forgetful in doing everyday activities such as running errands, doing chores, keeping appointments, returning phone calls, paying bills, etc.?

IF YES: What kinds of things do you frequently forget to do?
Is this the way you normally are?
Have you been this way most of your life?

IF EVIDENCE OF SYMPTOM: Were you like this as a child also? (Beginning at what age?)

A2. <u>Hyperactivity and impulsivity</u>: Five (or more) of the following symptoms have persisted for at least 6 months to a degree that is inconsistent with developmental level and that negatively impacts directly on social and academic/occupational activities.

1. Often fidgets with or taps hands or feet or squirms in seat.

Is it hard for you to sit still?
Are you fidgety?
Do you frequently tap your hands or shake your feet?

IF YES TO ANY: Is that the way you normally are?
Have you been this way most of your life?

IF EVIDENCE OF SYMPTOM: Were you like this as a child also? (Beginning at what age?)

2. Often leaves seat in situations when remaining seated is expected (e.g., in classroom, office, workplace, or other situations that require remaining seated).

Is it difficult for you to sit for a long time, even in situations in which you are expected to remain seated such as a classroom or meeting?

IF YES: Examples.
Is that the way you normally are?
Have you been this way most of your life?

IF EVIDENCE OF SYMPTOM: Were you like this as a child also? (Beginning at what age?)

3. Often runs about or climbs in situations where it is inappropriate (In adolescents or adults, may be limited to feeling restless).

Do you often feel restless inside?
IF YES: Is that the way you normally are?
Have you been this way most of your life?

IF EVIDENCE OF SYMPTOM: Were you like this as a child also? (Beginning at what age?) (Did you run about or climb things when it was inappropriate?)

4. Often unable to play or engage in leisure activities quietly.

Do you tend to be a loud and noisy person?
Do other people sometimes tell you to quiet down or lower your voice?
IF YES: In what types of situations?
IF YES TO EITHER: Is that the way you normally are?
Have you been this way most of your life?

IF EVIDENCE OF SYMPTOM: Were you like this as a child also? (Beginning at what age?)

5. Is often "on the go," acting as if "driven by a motor" (e.g., is unable to be or uncomfortable being still for an extended time, as in restaurants, meetings, etc.).

Are you constantly moving and on the go?
Is it hard to slow down or stop even when you want to?
Does it feel like there is a motor inside you that never shuts off?
IF YES TO ANY: Is that the way you normally are?
Have you been this way most of your life?

IF EVIDENCE OF SYMPTOM: Were you like this as a child also? (Beginning at what age?)

6. Often talks excessively.

Do you talk more than most people you know?
Has anyone ever commented on this or told you to stop talking?
IF YES TO EITHER: Is that the way you normally are?
Have you been this way most of your life?

IF EVIDENCE OF SYMPTOM: Were you like this as a child also? (Beginning at what age?)

7. Often blurts out an answer before a question has been completed (e.g., completes people's sentences; cannot wait for next turn in conversation).

Do you often answer someone's questions before they had a chance to finish asking it?
Do you often finish someone's sentence?
IF YES TO EITHER: Is that the way you normally are?
Have you been this way most of your life?

IF EVIDENCE OF SYMPTOM: Were you like this as a child also? (Beginning at what age?)

8. Often has difficulty waiting his or her turn (e.g., while waiting in line).

Is it difficult for you to wait in line?
More generally, is it hard for you to wait your turn when the situation calls for it?
IF YES TO EITHER: Is that the way you normally are?
Have you been this way most of your life?

IF EVIDENCE OF SYMPTOM: Were you like this as a child also? (Beginning at what age?)

9. Often interrupts or intrudes on others (e.g., butts into conversations, games, or activities; may start using other people's things without asking or receiving permission; takes over what others are doing).

Do you often interrupt people when they are busy or talking with others?
Do you butt into others' conversations?
Do you use others' things without permission because you can't wait to get their permission?
IF YES TO ANY: Is this the way you normally are?
Have you been this way most of your life?

IF EVIDENCE OF SYMPTOM: Were you like this as a child also? (Beginning at what age?)

(B) Several inattentive or hyperactive-impulsive symptoms were present prior to age 12.

IF AGE OF ONSET NOT ALREADY ESTABLISHED:
How old were you when you began [BEHAVIORS NOTED ABOVE]?

(C) Several symptoms are present in two or more settings (e.g., at home, school or work, with friends or relatives, or in other activities).

(D) There must be clear evidence that the symptoms interfere with or reduce the quality of social, academic, or occupational functioning.

IF IMPAIRMENT NOT ALREADY ESTABLISHED:
What problems do [BEHAVIORS NOTED ABOVE] cause?
Do [BEHAVIORS] bother other people? Do they cause problems at work? School? Home? In social relationships?

(E) Exclude the diagnosis if the symptoms occur exclusively during the course of Schizophrenia or another Psychotic Disorder and are not better accounted for by another mental disorder (e.g., Mood Disorder, Anxiety Disorder, Dissociative Disorder, Substance Use, or a Personality Disorder).

ATTENTION DEFICIT/HYPERACTIVITY DISORDER—Child

Inclusion: At least 6 from A1 or A2, B, C, D
Exclusion: E

A. EITHER A1 OR A2:

A1. Inattention: Six (or more) of the following symptoms have persisted for at least 6 months to a degree that is inconsistent with developmental level and that negatively impacts directly on social and academic/occupational activities.

Note: The interview questions in this section are written from the perspective of interviewing a child. The questions will need to be reworded if interviewing a parent about their child. Questions for assessing adults are on pages 85-89. The specific criteria are the same for adults and children.

1. Often fails to give close attention to details or makes careless mistakes in schoolwork, at work, or during other activities (e.g., overlooks or misses details, work is inaccurate).

Some kids have problems paying close attention to things, and because of this they make a lot of careless mistakes in their schoolwork. Is this something that you do?
IF YES: Does it happen a lot?
Has it affected your grades?

Do you often make careless mistakes when doing chores, or playing games? **IF YES:** Examples.

2. Often has difficulty sustaining attention in tasks or play activities (e.g., has difficulty remaining focused during lectures, conversations, or lengthy reading).

Some kids have a hard time keeping their mind on the thing they are doing because it is hard to pay attention to one thing for a long time. Is it hard for you to stay on track to only one thing for a long time?

Is it hard for you to stick with one thing, even when it's fun?

Is it hard to focus on a test or assignment that lasts an entire period?
IF YES TO ANY: Does your poor attention span cause problems?

3. Often does not seem to listen when spoken to directly (e.g., mind seems elsewhere, even in the absence of obvious distraction).

Do you often have problems focusing on what others say to you, even when they are speaking directly to you?
Have others commented that you don't seem to be listening?

Do your teachers say that you don't listen when they talk to you?
Do they have to ask you the same thing again before you hear them?

What about your parents? Do they often have to repeat what they say to you? Do they sometimes say you "must be deaf?"

4. Often does not follow through on instructions and fails to finish schoolwork, chores, or duties in the workplace (e.g., starts tasks but quickly loses focus and is easily sidetracked).

Some kids have difficulty completing things. Is that true of you?

What about chores around the house? Do you start doing them and leave in the middle?
IF YES: Do you do that a lot?
Is it hard to stick with it, or do you stop because you don't like doing the chore?

5. Often has difficulty organizing tasks and activities (e.g., difficulty managing sequential tasks; difficulty keeping materials and belongings in order; messy, disorganized work; poor time management; tends to fail to meet deadlines).

Is being organized difficult for you?
IF YES: Tell me about that.
Is it difficult for you to plan and organize your schoolwork?
IF YES: What happens?
Do you need your mom's or dad's help getting organized to do school projects?

Is your work space at school or home messy and disorganized?

Are you poor in managing your time?
Are you often late turning in assignments?
IF YES: Examples.

6. Often avoids, dislikes, or is reluctant to engage in tasks that require sustained mental effort (e.g., schoolwork or homework, preparing reports, completing forms, or reviewing lengthy papers).

Some kids really hate doing schoolwork or homework because it's hard for them to concentrate on it for a long time. Are you like that?

Do you often avoid or put off doing a task that requires a lot of concentration? Examples.

7. Often loses things necessary for tasks or activities (e.g., school materials, pencils, books, tools, wallets, keys, paperwork, eyeglasses, or mobile telephones).

Do you lose things a lot?
Do you frequently lose your pen, pencil, books, homework?
What about toys, keys, money? Do you lose them a lot?

8. Is often easily distracted by extraneous stimuli.

Is it difficult for you to keep your mind on the things you want to do because you are easily distracted?
IF YES: What kinds of things distract you?
How common is this?

9. Is often forgetful in daily activities (e.g., doing chores, running errands, keeping appointments).

Are you forgetful in doing everyday activities such as running errands, keeping appointments, doing chores?

Do you forget to do things like brushing your teeth, washing your hands, changing your underwear?
IF YES: Is this forgetfulness, or is it that you don't like doing these things?

A2. <u>Hyperactivity and impulsivity</u>: Six (or more) of the following symptoms have persisted for at least 6 months to a degree that is inconsistent with developmental level and that negatively impacts directly on social and academic/occupational activities.

Note: The symptoms are not solely a manifestation of oppositional behavior, defiance, hostility, or a failure to understand instructions.

1. Often fidgets with or taps hands or feet or squirms in seat.

Is it hard for you to sit still?
Is it hard to sit still while watching TV, playing a game, or doing homework, or while you're sitting in class at school?
Has anyone ever said that you can't seem to sit still, or that it seems like you have "ants in your pants?"

2. Often leaves seat in situations when remaining seated is expected (e.g., in classroom, office, workplace, or other situations that require remaining seated).

Is it difficult for you to stay in your seat in school?
Do you get out of your seat a lot when you're not supposed to?

Do you stay in your chair during all of breakfast or all of dinner, at home or in a restaurant, or do you get up a lot?

3. Often runs about or climbs in situations where it is inappropriate.

Do you run around the house or climb on furniture a lot?
Do you climb on desks or other things in school?
Do you jump down the stairs or run down the halls?
IF YES TO ANY:
Do your teachers/parents often have to tell you to stop running around so much?
Do you get into trouble for this?

4. Often unable to play or engage in leisure activities quietly.

Do your parents frequently tell you to quiet down when you play?
Are you noisier than other kids your age?
Is this a problem at school?

5. Is often "on the go," acting as if "driven by a motor" (e.g., is unable to be or uncomfortable being still for an extended time, as in restaurants, meetings, etc.).

Are you often on the go, doing something?
Are you more active than other kids your age?
Does it feel like there is a motor inside you that never shuts off?

6. Often talks excessively.

Do you talk a lot? **IF YES:** More than other kids?

Do your parents or teachers say that you're a chatterbox because you never stop talking?

7. Often blurts out an answer before a question has been completed (e.g., completes people's sentences; cannot wait for next turn in conversation).

When your teachers ask questions, do you tend to answer the question out loud before the teacher has a chance to finish asking it?
IF YES: How often does this happen?
Has your teacher spoken to you or your parents about this?

Do you often complete others' sentences when they are speaking?

8. Often has difficulty waiting his or her turn (e.g., while waiting in line).

For some kids it is hard for them to wait their turn when playing games. Is this hard for you?

Is it hard for you to wait in line in stores, or going to movies, or other activities where you have to wait in line?

When you eat with your family is it hard for you to wait to get served?
IF YES: Do others get upset with you because of this?

9. Often interrupts or intrudes on others (e.g., butts into conversations, games, or activities; may start using other people's things without asking or receiving permission; take over what others are doing).

Do your parents get angry at you because you interrupt them when they are busy or talking with others?

Do you often interrupt your parents when they are on the phone?

Do other kids tell you to leave them alone so they could do their work?
Do you butt into other kids' games before they ask you to play?

(B) Several inattentive or hyperactive-impulsive symptoms were present prior to age 12.

IF AGE OF ONSET NOT ALREADY ESTABLISHED:
How old were you when you began [BEHAVIORS NOTED ABOVE]?

(C) Several symptoms are present in two or more settings (e.g, at home, school or work, with friends or relatives, or in other activities).

(D) There must be clear evidence that the symptoms interfere with or reduce the quality of social, academic, or occupational functioning.

IF IMPAIRMENT NOT ALREADY ESTABLISHED:
What problems do [BEHAVIORS NOTED ABOVE] cause?
Do [BEHAVIORS] bother other people?
Do they cause problems at school? Home? With friends or classmates?

(E) <u>Exclude</u> the diagnosis if the symptoms occur exclusively during the course of Schizophrenia or another Psychotic Disorder and are not better accounted for by another mental disorder (e.g., Mood Disorder, Anxiety Disorder, Dissociative Disorder, Substance Use, or a Personality Disorder).

CONDUCT DISORDER

Inclusion: at least 3 from A, B
Exclusion: none

A. A repetitive and persistent pattern of behavior in which the basic rights of others or major age-appropriate societal norms or rules are violated, as manifested by the presence of 3 or more of the following 15 criteria in the past 12 months, with at least one criterion present in the past 6 months.

AGGRESSION TO PEOPLE AND ANIMALS

(A1) Often bullies, threatens, or intimidates others.

Do you pick on other kids?
IF YES: How often?

Do you pick on kids that are younger or smaller than you?
Are you a bully?

Do you ever threaten other kids so they will buy you things, give you money, or do other things for you?
IF YES: How often? Describe.

(A2) Often initiates physical fights.

Do you get into many fights? (More than other kids?)
IF YES: How often?
How often do you start the fights?

(A3) Has used a weapon that can cause serious physical harm to others (e.g., a bat, brick, broken bottle, knife, gun).

Have you ever used a weapon in a fight?
IF YES: What did you use?
For what reason?
How often did that happen?

(A4) Has been physically cruel to people.

Have you hurt people physically?
IF YES: What did you do to them? For what reason?

(A5) Has been physically cruel to animals.

Have you ever hurt, tortured, or killed an animal?
IF YES: What did you do?

Have you ever hurt a pet of yours?
IF YES: What did you do?

(A6) Has stolen while confronting a victim (e.g., mugging, purse snatching, extortion, armed robbery).

Have you ever taken things from people like snatching a purse, jewelry, or chains?

Have you ever held anyone up or mugged a person?

Have you ever robbed a store?
IF YES TO ANY: What did you do?

(A7) Has forced someone into sexual activity.

Have you ever forced anyone to have sex with you?
Were you ever part of a group or gang that forced someone to have sex against his/her will?
IF YES TO EITHER: What happened?

DESTRUCTION OF PROPERTY

(A8) Has deliberately engaged in fire setting with the intention of causing serious damage.

Have you ever set things on fire?
IF YES: For what reason?

(A9) Has deliberately destroyed others' property (other than by fire setting).

Have you ever deliberately damaged someone's property (e.g., breaking windows, spraying graffiti, etc.)?
IF YES: What did you do?

DECEITFULNESS OR THEFT

(A10) Has broken into someone else's house, building , or car.

Have you ever broken into someone's house, a store, building or car?
IF YES: For what reason?
Did you do it alone or with someone?

(A11) Often lies to obtain goods or favors or to avoid obligations (i.e., "cons" others).

Do you tell a lot of lies?
IF YES: Do you think you lie a lot or a little?

Do you often lie to get things that you wanted?

Do you often lie to avoid chores or responsibilities?

(A12) Has stolen items of nontrivial value without confronting a victim (e.g., shoplifting, burglary, forgery).

How often have you stolen from stores, your parents, or other people? (What did you steal? What's the most you have stolen?)

Did you ever get caught stealing?
IF YES: What happened?

Did you ever pick someone's pocket, write a forged check, or use a credit card without permission? **IF YES:** What did you do?

SERIOUS VIOLATIONS OF THE RULES

(A13) Often stays out all night despite parental prohibitions, beginning before age 13.

Do you argue with your parents about how late you can stay out at night?

How often have you stayed out all night when they said you couldn't?
IF PRESENT: How old were you when you first did this?

(A14) Has run away from home overnight at least twice while living in parental or parental surrogate home (or once without returning for a lengthy period).

Did you ever run away from home overnight?
IF YES: How often?
How long did you stay away?

(A15) Is often truant from school, beginning before age 13.

How often have you played hooky or skipped school?
IF PRESENT: How old were you the first time you skipped school?

(B) The disturbance in behavior causes significant impairment in social, academic, or occupational functioning.

What problems have [BEHAVIORS] caused?

Has it caused problems at school? (Suspension? Expulsion?)

Has it affected your friendships or family life?

Have you gotten into legal problems?

OPPOSITIONAL DEFIANT DISORDER

Inclusion: at least 4 from A, B
Exclusion: C

NOTE: For each symptom you must determine whether it is present more than most boys/girls the child's age. For children under age 5, the behavior should occur on most days for at least 6 months (except criterion A8). For children 5 years or older, the behavior should occur at least once per week for at least 6 months (except A8).

NOTE: Because the disorder is more common in boys than girls, and the diagnosis is usually based on parental report, the questions are written as if a parent is being interviewed about his/her son.

A. A pattern of angry/irritable mood, argumentative/defiant behavior, or vindictiveness lasting at least six months as evidenced by 4 or more symptoms from any of the following categories, observed during interaction with at least one individual who is not a sibling.

(A1) Often loses temper.

Does [SON] have a bad temper? **IF YES:** Tell me about that.
Does he have temper tantrums?
IF YES: What causes them? How often does he have them?

(A2) Is often touchy or easily annoyed.

Does he easily get annoyed by others?
Is he hypersensitive and quick to react with anger?

(A3) Is often angry and resentful.

Does he seem to be angry a lot of the time?
Is he easily bothered by other people telling him what to do?
IF YES: Examples.
Does he often complain that he is not being treated fairly?

(A4) Often argues with authority figures or adults.

Does he frequently argue with you or [SPOUSE]?
IF YES: About what?
Does he always find something to argue about?
Does he frequently argue with teachers or other adults?
IF YES: Like who? About what?

(A5) Often actively defies or refuses to comply with requests from authority figures or rules.

Does he have trouble following rules?
Does he seem to break the rules on purpose?
IF YES TO EITHER: Tell me about that.
Does he often say no when you or teachers ask him to do something?
IF YES: Examples.

(A6) Often deliberately annoys others.

Does he like to do things that annoy or bother other people?
IF YES: Like what? How often does he do things like that?

(A7) Often blames others for his or her mistakes or misbehavior.

Is it hard for him to admit that he is wrong when he made a mistake?
Does he blame others for his mistakes?
Does he blame others when he misbehaves or gets into trouble?

(A8) Has been spiteful or vindictive at least twice in the past six months.

When he feels he is wronged does he try to get back at the other person?
IF YES: What has he done?
How often does he do things like this?
(When was the last time?)

(B) The disturbance in behavior is associated with distress in the individual or others in his or her immediate social context (e.g., family, peer group, work colleagues) or it impacts negatively on social, educational, occupation or other areas of functioning.

What problems have [BEHAVIORS] caused?
Has it caused problems at school? (Suspension? Transfer?)
Has it caused him to lose friends?
What about problems at home?

(C) <u>Exclude</u> the diagnosis if the symptoms occur exclusively during the course of a Psychotic, Substance Use, Depressive, or Bipolar Disorder. Also the individual does not meet criteria for Disruptive Mood Dysregulation Disorder.

SEPARATION ANXIETY DISORDER

Inclusion: At least 3 from A, B, C
Exclusion: D

A. Developmentally inappropriate and excessive fear or anxiety concerning separation from those to whom the individual is attached, as evidenced by 3 or more of the following:

(A1) Recurrent excessive distress when anticipating or experiencing separation from home or major attachment figures.

(MAF = Major Attachment Figure, i.e. parent, sibling, child)

Do you worry a lot about being away from your MAF?

Do you get anxious when you're away from home?

(A2) Persistent and excessive worry about losing major attachment figures or possible harm to them, such as illness, injury, disasters, or death.

Do you worry a lot that something bad will happen to your MAF?
Do you worry a lot that they will get sick or hurt?
Do you often get scared that they will die or be taken from you?
IF YES TO ANY:
Why are you scared about that?
For how long have you been worrying about that?

(A3) Persistent and excessive worry about experiencing an untoward event (e.g., getting lost, being kidnapped, having an accident, dying) that cause separation from a major attachment figure.

Do you get scared a lot about getting lost and separated from your MAF when you leave the house?

Do you get scared that you will be kidnapped, and you would never see your MAF again?
IF YES: How often do you worry that ____________?
For how long have you been worrying about this?

(A4) Persistent reluctance or refusal to go out, away from home, to school, work, or elsewhere because of fear of separation.

Are you reluctant, or do you refuse, to leave the house because of discomfort about being away from your MAF?

(For example, when you first started going to school was it hard for you to go because you didn't want to be away from your MAF?)
IF YES: Did they have to drag you to school?
Did you refuse to go?

(A5) Persistent and excessive fear or reluctance about being alone or without major attachment figures at home or in other settings.

Is it scary for you to be alone at home?

Are there places outside of the house where you feel uncomfortable when you're alone without your MAF?

(A6) Persistent reluctance or refusal to sleep away from home or to go to sleep without being near a major attachment figure.

Do you sleep alone or with your MAF?
Are you afraid of going to sleep alone?
Is it hard to sleep when your MAF isn't around?
Do you sometimes not go to sleep until your MAF is in the house?

Are you allowed to sleep at someone else's house?
IF YES: Have you ever been invited to stay at someone's house?
IF YES: Did you go?
IF NO: Why not?
IF YES: How was it being away from your MAF?

(A7) Repeated nightmares involving the theme of separation.

Do you have a lot of scary dreams or nightmares?
IF YES: What are they about?
Do you have any nightmares about being separated from your MAF—like being kidnapped or your MAF going away?

(A8) Repeated complaints of physical symptoms (e.g., headaches, stomachaches, nausea, or vomiting) when anticipating or experiencing separation from major attachment figures.

Do you get physically sick when you are not with your MAF?
Do you often get sick before you go to school or work in the morning?
Do you get physically sick just thinking about your MAF golng somewhere without you?

IF YES TO ANY: What physical symptoms do you get?
How often does this happen?

(B) The fear, anxiety or avoidance is persistent, typically lasting 4 weeks in children and adolescents (and 6 or more months in adults).

IF NOT CLEAR FROM ABOVE INFORMATION:
For how long have you [SYMPTOMS NOTED ABOVE]?

(C) The disturbance causes clinically significant distress or impairment in social, academic, occupational, or other important areas of functioning.

What problems have the [BEHAVIORS NOTED ABOVE] caused?
Have your grades suffered or have you missed a lot of school?
Have you missed a lot of work?
Has it affected the number of friends you have?

(D) Exclude the diagnosis if the anxiety is better accounted for by another mental disorder (e.g., refusing to leave home in Autism Spectrum Disorder; delusions or hallucinations concerning separation in Psychotic Disorders; anxiety about having panic attacks in Panic Disorder or agoraphobia situations in Agoraphobia; ill health in Generalized Anxiety Disorder; having an illness in Illness Anxiety Disorder; or separation from attachment figures due to trauma in Posttraumatic Stress Disorder).

Personality Disorders

PARANOID PERSONALITY DISORDER

Inclusion: at least 4 from A
Exclusion: B

A. A pervasive distrust and suspiciousness of others such that their motives are interpreted as malevolent, beginning by early adulthood and present in a variety of contexts, as indicated by 4 or more of the following:

(A1) Suspects, without sufficient basis, that others are exploiting, harming, or deceiving him or her.

Have you had experiences where people who pretended to be your friends took advantage of you?
IF YES: What happened? How often has this happened?

Are you good at spotting someone trying to deceive or con you?
IF YES: How can you tell?

Are you concerned that someone might be trying to hurt you?
IF YES: Tell me about that.

(A2) Is preoccupied with unjustified doubts about the loyalty or trustworthiness of friends or associates.

Are you concerned that certain friends or coworkers are not really loyal or trustworthy?
IF YES: How much time do you think about this?
What has caused your concern?
Has this made your life difficult?

(A3) Is reluctant to confide in others because of unwarranted fear that the information will be used maliciously against him or her.

Some people are very reluctant to confide in other people. Are you like this?
IF YES: Why is that?

Do you usually find there's a price to pay when you've shared something personal with others?
IF YES: Does this keep you from opening up to others?
What might happen if you did confide?

(A4) Reads hidden demeaning or threatening meanings into benign remarks or events.

Do people frequently seem to do things just to annoy you?
IF YES: Like what?

Do you usually take what people tell you at face value, or do you frequently try to figure out what they really mean?
IF FIGURE OUT:
What kinds of things do you think they really mean?
Are their comments often hidden threats or put downs?

(A5) Persistently bears grudges, i.e., is unforgiving of insults, injuries, or slights.

How long would you stay angry at someone who does something to hurt or insult you like not inviting you to a party?
Do you tend to hold grudges?
How long does it take you to forgive someone who insults you?

(A6) Perceives attacks on his/her character or reputation that are not apparent to others and is quick to react angrily or counterattack.

Do people say things to attack you or ruin your reputation, even though it might not seem that way to others?
IF YES: Tell me about that. How do you react to this?

Do you find that people often make indirect comments to attack you or put you down, rather than tell you directly?
IF YES: How do you react? Do you get angry?
Do you try to get back at the person?

Do other people say that you read too much into things and take offense at things that were not meant to be critical?

(A7) Has recurrent suspicions, without justification, regarding fidelity of spouse or sexual partner.

When you've been involved in a relationship, do you often worry that your partner is unfaithful to you?
IF YES: What causes your concerns? How did it turn out?

(B) <u>Exclude</u> the diagnosis if the features only occurred during the course of Schizophrenia, a Mood Disorder with Psychotic Features, or another Psychotic Disorder, and are not due to the direct physiological effects of a general medical condition.

SCHIZOID PERSONALITY DISORDER

Inclusion: at least 4 from A
Exclusion: B

A. A pervasive pattern of detachment from social relationships and a restricted range of expression of emotions in interpersonal settings, beginning by early adulthood and present in a variety of contexts, as indicated by 4 or more of the following:

(A1) Neither desires nor enjoys close relationships, including being part of a family.

Do you have any close relationships with friends or family?
IF YES: With whom?
What do you enjoy about these relationships?
IF NO: Does this bother you?
Do you wish you had some close relationships?

(A2) Almost always chooses solitary activities.

Some people prefer to spend time with other people, while others prefer to work and do things alone. How would you describe yourself?
IF ALONE: Do you almost always choose to do things by yourself?

(A3) Has little, if any, interest in having sexual experiences with another person.

In general, has your sex life been important to you, or could you have gotten along as well without it?
IF NOT IMPORTANT OR NOT CURRENTLY INVOLVED:
Would it bother you to live your entire life without sexual relationships?

(A4) Takes pleasure in few, if any, activities.

What kinds of activities do you enjoy?
IF ONLY 1 OR 2 ARE MENTIONED:
If [ACTIVITIES MENTIONED] were not available, are there any other things you would enjoy doing?

(A5) Lacks close friends or confidants other than first-degree relatives.

Not counting your immediate family, do you have any close friends you can confide in?

(A6) Appears indifferent to the praise or criticism of others.

How do you react when someone criticizes you?
IF NO REACTION: So you don't look or feel upset after you are criticized?

How do you react when someone compliments you?
IF NO REACTION: So you don't smile or think about it later and feel good about it?

(A7) Shows emotional coldness, detachment, or flattened affectivity.

[NOTE OBSERVATIONS]

[Is he/she slow to look you in the eye when talking?]
[Does he/she usually smile or nod back at you during conversation?]
[Can you tell what he/she is feeling by the expression on his/her face?]

(B) Exclude the diagnosis if the features only occurred during the course of Schizophrenia, a Mood Disorder with Psychotic Features, or another Psychotic Disorder, and are not due to the direct physiological effects of a general medical condition.

SCHIZOTYPAL PERSONALITY DISORDER

Inclusion: at least 5 from A
Exclusion: B

A. A pervasive pattern of social and interpersonal deficits marked by acute discomfort with, and reduced capacity for, close relationships as well as by cognitive or perceptual distortions and eccentricities of behavior, beginning by early adulthood and present in a variety of contexts, as indicated by 5 or more of the following:

(A1) Ideas of reference (excluding delusions of reference).

Have you ever found that people around you seem to be talking in general, but then you realize their comments are really meant for you?
IF YES: How do you know they are talking about you?

When you walk into a room, does is sometimes seem like people stop talking or act differently?
IF YES: How often does this happen?

Have you ever noticed that someone in charge changed the rules specifically because of you, but they wouldn't admit it?

Do you sometimes feel like strangers on the street are looking at you or talking about you?
IF YES: Why do you think they notice you in particular?

(A2) Odd beliefs or magical thinking, that influence behavior and are inconsistent with subcultural norms (i.e., superstitiousness, belief in clairvoyance, telepathy, or "sixth sense;" in children and adolescents, bizarre fantasies or preoccupations).

A number of people talk about having telepathy or ESP and feel like they can sense what's in someone's mind or predict the future. Have you had any experiences like this?
IF YES: How often? Are these experiences important to you?
IF YES: How? Have your friends and family also had experiences like this?

Are you a superstitious person?
IF YES: In what way?
How does this influence your decisions or behavior?
Do your friends and family share these superstitions?

Some people believe they can influence things like the weather or ball games just by thinking about them. Do you believe that you can make things happen just by thinking about them?
IF YES: Tell me about that.

Do you believe in hexes, curses, omens, voodoo, witchcraft, magic, or other things like that?
IF YES: Tell me about that.
How does this influence your decisions or behavior?
Do your friends and family share these beliefs?

(A3) Unusual perceptual experiences, including bodily illusions.

Have you ever sensed there was some unusual force or presence in the room?
IF YES: Can you describe what this was like?
What do you think causes this?
How often has this happened?

Have you ever felt like the world around you looked different than it usually does?
Have colors or shapes ever seemed changed or different than normal?
IF YES TO EITHER: What was this like?
Were you using drugs or alcohol at the time?

Do your eyes ever play tricks on you—for instance, someone's face or body seems to change in shape or form?
IF YES: Can you describe what this was like?

Do you ever mistake noises for voices, or shadows or objects for people?
IF YES: How often does this happen?

(A4) Odd thinking and speech (e.g., vague, circumstantial, metaphorical, overelaborate, or stereotyped).

[NOTE OBSERVATIONS]
[Does he/she seem to talk in an odd or unusual way?]
IF YES: How so?
[When he/she talks about something, do you find it hard to follow what he/she is saying?]

(A5) Suspiciousness or paranoid ideation.

Have you had experiences where people who pretended to be your friends took advantage of you?
IF YES: What happened?
How often has this happened?

Do you often worry that people might be planning to harm or take advantage of you?
IF YES: Why do you think that?

Are you reluctant to confide in others because the information might be used against you?
IF YES: What caused this concern?

Do you usually take what people tell you at face value, or do you frequently try to figure out what they really mean?
IF FIGURE OUT:
What kinds of things do you think they really mean?
Do the comments often turn out to be hidden threats or put downs?

Do other people say that you read too much into things and take offense at things that were not meant to be critical?
IF YES: Example?

(A6) Inappropriate or constricted affect.

[NOTE OBSERVATIONS]
[Is there anything peculiar about the way he/she shows his/her emotions?]
[Does it seem like he/she never expresses any emotion?]
[Does he/she often laugh or smile for no good reason?]
[Does it often seem like the emotion he/she is showing does not fit with what he/she is saying?]

(A7) Behavior or appearance that is odd, eccentric, or peculiar.

[NOTE OBSERVATIONS]

[Is there anything odd or peculiar about the way he/she looks?
[Does he/she dress in an odd or peculiar way that is not explained by current fashion trends?

IF YES: Do you think he/she dresses this way to attract attention?
(RATING NOTE: SCHIZOTYPES GENERALLY DO NOT DRESS TO GET ATTENTION.)

[Does he/she do odd or peculiar things?]
[Does he/she often talk to himself/herself?]

(A8) Lacks close friends or confidants other than first-degree relatives.

Not counting your immediate family, do you have any close friends you can confide in?

(A9) Excessive social anxiety that does not diminish with familiarity and tends to be associated with paranoid fears rather than negative judgments about self.

Do you generally feel nervous or anxious around people?

IF YES: How bad does it get?
What makes you nervous?
Do you get nervous around people because you are worried about what they might do to you, or are you nervous because you don't feel you're as good as other people?
Are you less nervous after you get to know people better?

(B) Exclude the diagnosis if the features only occurred during the course of Schizophrenia, a Mood Disorder with Psychotic Features, or another Psychotic Disorder, and are not due to the direct physiological effects of a general medical condition.

BORDERLINE PERSONALITY DISORDER

Inclusion: at least 5 criteria
Exclusion: None

A pervasive pattern of instability of interpersonal relationships, self-image, and affects, and marked impulsivity beginning by early adulthood and present in a variety of contexts, as indicated by 5 or more of the following:

(1) Frantic efforts to avoid real or imagined abandonment. [Do not include suicidal or self-mutilating behavior covered in criterion 5].

Have there been times when you've been very upset, almost to the point of being distraught, because you thought someone you loved or needed very much might leave you?
IF YES: How often has this happened?
What did you do to keep them from leaving?
IF ONLY SUICIDAL/SELF-MUTILATING BEHAVIOR:
What else have you done?

Do you spend a lot of time thinking about ways to keep people from leaving you?

(2) A pattern of unstable and intense interpersonal relationships characterized by alternating between extremes of idealization and devaluation.

Do your relationships with friends and lovers tend to be intense and stormy with lots of ups and downs?
IF YES: Can you tell me about some of them?

With some people do you switch from loving, respecting, and admiring them at one time, to despising them at another time?
IF YES: Tell me about that.

(3) Identity disturbance: markedly and persistently unsteady self-image or sense of self.

Does the way you think about yourself change so often that you don't know who you are? **IF YES:** Tell me about this.

Do you ever feel like you're someone else, or that you're evil, or maybe that you don't even exist? **IF YES:** Tell me about that.

(4) Impulsivity in at least two areas that are potentially self-damaging (e.g., spending, sex, substance abuse, reckless driving, binge eating). NOTE: DO NOT INCLUDE SUICIDAL OR SELF-MUTILATING BEHAVIOR COVERED IN CRITERION 5.

I am going to ask you about some behaviors that sometimes cause problems for people. How many times in the past 5 years have you…

a) gambled more money than you could afford to lose?
b) spent money impulsively on things you didn't need or couldn't afford?
c) had one night stands or brief sexual affairs?
d) been intoxicated with alcohol?
e) been stoned or high on other drugs?
f) shoplifted or took something that didn't belong to you?
g) been in an auto accident, received a speeding ticket, or been charged with reckless driving?
h) driven while intoxicated or high?
i) gone on eating binges (ate a large amount of food in a short time and felt like you lost control of your eating)?
j) done anything else impulsive where you could have gotten hurt?

(5) Recurrent suicidal behavior, gestures, or threats, or self-mutilating behavior.

Have you ever been so upset that you told someone that you wanted to hurt or kill yourself?

IF YES: Tell me about that.
How often have you done this?

Have you ever made a suicide attempt, even one that wasn't very serious?

IF YES: What did you do?
How many attempts have you made?

Have you ever been so upset or tense that you deliberately hurt yourself by cutting your skin, putting your hand through a glass window, punching a wall, burning yourself, or anything else like that?

IF YES: What have you done?
How often?

(6) Affective instability due to a marked reactivity of mood (e.g., intense episodic dysphoria, irritability, or anxiety usually lasting a few hours and only rarely more than a few days).

Has anyone ever told you that your moods seem to change a great deal?
IF YES: What did they say?

Do you often have days when your mood changes a great deal—days when you shift back and forth from feeling like your usual self, to feeling angry or depressed or anxious?
IF YES: How intense are your mood swings?
How often does this happen in a typical week?
How long do the moods last?

(7) Chronic feelings of emptiness.

Do you feel empty much of the time?
IF YES: What percent of the time do you feel this way?

(8) Inappropriate, intense anger or difficulty controlling anger (e.g., frequent displays of temper, constant anger, recurrent physical fights).

How easily do you lose your temper?
How often do you lose your temper?

Do you feel angry much of the time?
What kinds of things get you really angry?
Are you sometimes angry without knowing why you feel that way?

Tell me what you are like when you are angry.
How long do you usually stay angry?

Do you ever throw or break things? Have you ever hit anyone? Do you get into physical fights?
IF YES TO ANY: Tell me about it.

When you are angry, do you ever give someone the silent treatment?
IF YES: For how long can you keep it up?
Is that a common reaction for you?

(9) Transient, stress-related paranoid ideation or severe dissociative symptoms.

When some people are under stress, they may have experiences that are very hard to explain to others. Have you ever felt like things around you were somehow strange, or changed in size or shape?

IF YES: Describe what that is like.

When you've been under stress, have you ever felt like your body or a part of it was somehow changed or not real?

Have you ever felt like you were watching yourself from outside your body?

IF YES: Describe what that was like.

Do you ever have brief blackouts and forget what has happened?

When you're feeling stressed, do you ever get paranoid or suspicious of people you usually trust?

IF NO: What about being afraid that someone is spying on you or planning to hurt you?

IF YES TO EITHER: Does this happen even when you're not stressed?

IF ANY OF THE ABOVE ARE POSITIVE, ASK:

You've said that you (LIST DISSOCIATIVE OR PARANOID EXPERIENCES): Were you using drugs or alcohol when this happened?

IF YES: Does this happen only when you're using drugs or alcohol?

IF OCCURS WHEN NOT USING DRUGS OR ALCOHOL:

How long do these experiences last?
Do they go away when you're not under stress?

ANTISOCIAL PERSONALITY DISORDER

Inclusion: A, at least 3 from B, at least 3 from C
Exclusion: D

A. Current age at least 18 years.

B. Evidence of Conduct Disorder with onset before age 15 as demonstrated by 3 or more of the following:

(B1) Often bullies, threatens or intimidates others.

As a child or teenager, did you pick on other kids?
IF YES: How often did this happen?

Did you pick on kids who were younger or smaller than you?
IF YES: Describe.

(B2) Often initiates physical fights.

Did you get into many fights? (More than other kids?)
IF YES: How often? How often did you start the fights?

(B3) Has used a weapon that can cause serious physical harm to others (e.g., a bat, brick, broken bottle, knife, gun).

Did you ever use a weapon in a fight?
IF YES: What did you use? For what reason?
How often did that happen?

(B4) Has stolen with confrontation with a victim (e.g., mugging, purse snatching, extortion, armed robbery).

As a child or teenager, did you ever take things from people like snatching a purse, jewelry, or chains?

Did you ever hold anyone up, or rob a store?

Did you ever threaten anyone if they didn't give you money?

(B5) Has been physically cruel to people.

Did you hurt people when you weren't in a fight?
IF YES: What did you do to them?
For what reason?

(B6) Has been physically cruel to animals.

Did you ever hurt or kill an animal?
IF YES: What did you do?

(B7) Has forced someone into sexual activity.

Did you ever force anyone to have sex with you?

Were you ever part of a group or gang that forced someone to have sex against his/her will?
IF YES: Tell me about that.

(B8) Often lies or breaks promises to obtain goods or favors or to avoid obligations (e.g., "cons" others).

Did you tell a lot of lies?
IF YES: For what reasons?
Did you often lie to get things that you wanted?

(B9) Often stays out at night, despite parental prohibitions, beginning before 13 years of age.

Did you argue with your parents about how late you could stay out at night?

Did you often stay out later than they said you could?

Did you ever stay out all night?
IF YES: How old were you when you first began doing this?

(B10) Has stolen items of nontrivial value without confrontation with the victim either within the home or outside the home (e.g., shoplifting, burglary, forgery).

As a child or teenager, did you steal from stores, your parents, or other people?
IF YES: What did you steal?
How often did you steal?

Did you ever pick someone's pocket, write a forged check, use a credit card or charge something online without permission?

(B11) Has deliberately engaged in fire setting with the intention of causing serious damage.

Did you ever set fires?
IF YES: Why?

(B12) Has deliberately destroyed other's property (other than by fire setting).

Did you damage someone's property by breaking windows, spraying graffiti on walls, or other things like that?
IF YES: What did you do?

(B13) Has run away from home overnight at least twice while living in parental or parental surrogate home (or once without returning for a lengthy period).

Did you ever run away from home overnight?
IF YES: How often?
How long did you stay away?

(B14) Often truant from school, beginning before 13 years of age.

Did you ever skip school?
IF YES: How many times did you do this?
Did you get into trouble for it?
How old were you (in what grade were you) when you started to skip school?

(B15) Has broken into someone else's home, building, or car.

Did you ever break into anyone's house, a store, building or car?

C. A pervasive pattern of disregard for and violation of the rights of others occurring since age 15, as indicated by 3 or more of the following:

(C1) Failure to conform to social norms with respect to lawful behavior as indicated by repeatedly performing acts that are grounds for arrest.

I am not interested in knowing any specific details that might get you in trouble, but I need to ask how many times you might have done any of the following in the last five years:

_____bought or sold stolen property
_____embezzled other people's money
_____ran numbers
_____sold drugs
_____shoplifted or stole things
_____had sex for money
_____hacked an online account
_____did other things that could have gotten you arrested

Have you ever been arrested?
IF YES: How many times?
What were the circumstances?

(C2) Irritability and aggressiveness, as indicated by repeated physical fights or assaults.

How often have you been in physical fights?

What about attacking or hitting someone?

Have you ever been so angry that you started throwing things at your spouse/partner?
IF YES: How often has this happened?

Have you ever spanked or hit a child hard enough so that he or she had bruises, had to stay in bed, or see a doctor?
IF YES: How many times has this happened?

(C3) Consistent irresponsibility, as indicated by repeated failure to sustain consistent work behavior or honor financial obligations.

Have you sometimes been unable to pay for household necessities such as food, rent, or the electric bill because you spent so much money on things you could have done without?

Have you sometimes not paid bills or other financial obligations?
IF YES: What were the circumstances?

Have you ever failed to make court ordered payments such as child support, alimony, or a lawsuit settlement?
IF YES: Tell me about it.

When you have been working, have you ever gotten into trouble for not arriving on time, missing too many days, not doing your work, or not following the rules?
IF YES: Tell me about it.

(C4) Impulsivity or failure to plan ahead.

How often have you just walked off a job or quit without any other work in sight? ("OTHER WORK" INCLUDES FULL-TIME STUDENT, HOMEMAKER, ETC.)
IF YES: Tell me about it.

How often have you impulsively picked up and moved around from place to place without any idea of how long you were going to stay or where you would go next?
IF YES: Tell me about it.

How often have you spent money impulsively on things you didn't need or couldn't afford?

Do you often get into trouble because you don't plan ahead?
IF YES: Examples?

(C5) Deceitfulness, as indicated by repeated lying, use of aliases, or conning others for personal profit or pleasure.

Is it easy for you to lie if it serves your purpose?

Have you ever used a false name or developed a scheme to con people into giving you what you want?

(C6) Reckless disregard for safety of self or others.

How often have you been in an auto accident?
IF MORE THAN ONE: How did they happen?

How often have you received speeding tickets or been charged with reckless driving?

What about driving while you were high on drugs or alcohol?

Are you known as someone who risks life and limb in recreational activities?
IF YES: How did you get this reputation?
IF NOT CLEARLY RECKLESS:
Do you take all recommended safety precautions when doing these things?

Did you ever get into trouble at work for doing things that could be dangerous to you or others?
IF YES: What happened?

(C7) Lack of remorse, as indicated by being indifferent to, or rationalizing having hurt, mistreated, or stolen from another.

You mentioned that you have [ANTISOCIAL BEHAVIOR(S) PREVIOUSLY DESCRIBED]. How do you feel about that?
IF NO REMORSE:
Do you ever feel sorry or guilty?
Do you think that [ANTISOCIAL BEHAVIOR(S) was justified?

D. <u>Exclude</u> the diagnosis if the occurrence of antisocial behavior is exclusively during the course of Schizophrenia or a Manic Episode.

NARCISSISTIC PERSONALITY DISORDER

Inclusion: at least 5 criteria
Exclusion: None

A pervasive pattern of grandiosity (in fantasy or behavior), need for admiration, and lack of empathy, beginning by early adulthood and present in a variety of contexts, as indicated by 5 or more of the following:

(1) Has a grandiose sense of self-importance (e.g., exaggerates achievements and talents, expects to be recognized as superior without commensurate achievements).

Would you describe yourself as someone who has or will accomplish great things—accomplishments that will set you apart from your equals?
IF YES: Tell me about them.

Have people told you that you have too high an opinion of yourself?
IF YES: Why do think they said that?

(2) Is preoccupied with fantasies of unlimited success, power, brilliance, beauty, or ideal love.

When people imagine what their life would be like if they could have anything they want, they may think of such things as power, success, brilliance, beauty, the perfect relationship, or other things. What do you daydream about? How often do you daydream about this?

Do your daydreams sometimes occupy your thoughts so much that it is hard to concentrate on your work or get things done?

How often do you feel bad or like a failure because you haven't achieved your dreams?

(3) Believes that he or she is "special" and unique and can only be understood by, or should associate with, other special or high-status people (or institutions).

Some people are so creative, intelligent, and unique that they have a hard time finding people like themselves to share things with. Does this sound like you?

IF YES: What kind of person is able to understand you and be a good friend?

Do you consider yourself a particularly special or unique person?

IF YES: In what way?
Have you always felt this way about yourself?
How has it affected how you relate to people?

Is it hard for others to understand you?

IF YES: Why is that?

(4) Requires excessive admiration.

Is the praise and admiration of friends and colleagues important to you?

IF YES: Do you often feel empty and hurt because people don't give you the praise and admiration you feel you deserve?

Has anyone ever accused you of fishing for compliments?

(5) Has a sense of entitlement, i.e., unreasonable expectations of especially favorable treatment or automatic compliance with his or her expectations.

Some people have earned the right to special consideration because of who they are, what they've done, or what they've gone through. Are there ways in which this applies to you?

IF YES: Tell me about that.

Do you often get angry or irritated because you don't get the treatment you think you deserve?

IF YES: Examples?

IF NO: Has anyone else ever said that you acted this way?

IF YES: What do you think made them say that?

Do you have a reputation for expecting others to do whatever you say without questioning?

(6) Is interpersonally exploitive, i.e., takes advantage of others to achieve his or her own ends.

Are you pretty good at getting people to do what you want?
IF YES: How do you get them to do what you want?
Do you ever pretend you're interested in someone so they'll do something for you? **IF YES:** How often?

Have you ever taken advantage of someone because it was the only way to get what you needed or deserved?
IF YES: Can you describe a situation?
How often have you done something like this?

Do you have a reputation for doing whatever it takes to get what you want, even if it means stepping on other people?

(7) Lacks empathy: is unwilling to recognize or identify with the feelings and needs of others.

How do you feel when others start telling you about their problems?

Is it hard for you to put yourself in someone else's shoes and understand what they're going through?
IF YES: Has this caused any problems for you?
Do you think you should try and understand?

Have other people complained that you are not very sympathetic to their problems?
IF YES: Why do you think they said that?

(8) Is often envious of others or believes that others are envious of him or her.

Are there people you really envy or are jealous of?
IF YES: What do you envy about them?
How often do you think about this?
Do you feel like you deserve what they have more than they do?
Does thinking about what they have bother you a lot or keep you from getting things done?

Are people often jealous or envious of you?
IF YES: Why do you think they're jealous?

(9) Shows arrogant, haughty behaviors or attitudes.

Have other people complained that you have an attitude problem?
IF YES: What do you think they mean?
What did they say?

Has anyone ever said that you act is if you have "a chip on your shoulder?"
IF YES: Why do you think they said that?

Has anyone ever said that you act in an arrogant way?
IF YES: Tell me about that.
How often has this occurred?
What problems has this caused?

(ALSO CONSIDER BEHAVIOR DURING THE INTERVIEW)

HISTRIONIC PERSONALITY DISORDER

Inclusion: at least 5 criteria
Exclusion: None

A pervasive pattern of excessive emotionality and attention seeking, beginning by early adulthood and present in a variety of contexts, as indicated by 5 or more of the following:

(1) Is uncomfortable in situations in which he or she is not the center of attention.

Some people prefer to be the center of attention while others are content to remain on the edge of things. Where would you put yourself?
IF CENTER: How do you feel when you're not the center of attention?

Have other people said that you always need to be the center of attention?

(2) Interaction with others is often characterized by inappropriate sexually seductive or provocative behavior.

Do you have a reputation for being a flirt?
IF YES: Tell me about that.

Do people sometimes misinterpret your friendliness as a romantic or sexual invitation?
IF YES: How often does that happen?

(ALSO CONSIDER BEHAVIOR DURING THE INTERVIEW).

(3) Displays rapidly shifting and shallow expression of emotions.

Do your emotions and feelings change quickly?
IF YES: Do other people notice?
Have you always been like that?

Has anyone ever commented that your emotions do not seem real or sincere?
IF YES: Tell me about that.

(ALSO CONSIDER BEHAVIOR DURING THE INTERVIEW).

(4) Consistently uses physical appearances to draw attention to self.

Compared to other people your age, are you more interested in having your appearance noticed?

How often do you use your appearance to get people's attention?
IF YES: How do you do that?

Are you disappointed when people don't notice how you look?

(ALSO CONSIDER APPEARANCE AND BEHAVIOR DURING THE INTERVIEW).

(5) Has a style of speech that is excessively impressionistic and lacking in detail.

(***NOTE THROUGHOUT THE INTERVIEW WHETHER THE INDIVIDUAL IS ABLE TO GIVE CONCRETE EXAMPLES WITH APPROPRIATE DETAIL, ESPECIALLY WHEN HE/SHE EXPRESSES A STRONG OPINION***)

(6) Shows self-dramatizatlon, theatricality, and exaggerated expression of emotion.

Some people are very expressive. They cry at weddings, embrace people, show their fear and their joy. Would you say you are more or less likely than most people to show your emotions?
IF MORE: Has this ever caused you problems or embarrassment?

Has anyone ever said anything about how you show your emotions?
IF YES: What did they say?
Do you agree?

Do you think you would make a good actor/actress?
IF YES: Why do you say that?

(ALSO CONSIDER EMOTIONAL EXPRESSIVITY DURING THE INTERVIEW)

(7) Is suggestible, i.e., easily influenced by others or circumstances.

Some people are so strongly influenced by others that they are easily swayed by their opinions. Do your opinions change easily depending on who you are with?

IF YES: How often does this happen?

Are you quick to adopt current fads and then give them up when they are no longer popular?

IF YES: Example.

If someone says they have a problem such as a headache or upset stomach, or they feel some strong emotion, do you suddenly feel the same way?

IF YES: Example.

(8) Considers relationships to be more intimate than they actually are.

Do you often feel a close bond to someone you have just met?

IF YES: Does this happen a lot?

Do you sometimes get hurt in relationships because you think the relationship is more serious than the other person does?

Are you quick to share personal details of your life with someone you have just met?

IF YES: Can you think of times when this was a problem?

Do you often feel a close personal relationship with bosses or professionals you haven't known very long?

OBSESSIVE-COMPULSIVE PERSONALITY DISORDER

Inclusion: at least 4 criteria
Exclusion: None

A pervasive pattern of preoccupation with orderliness, perfectionism, and mental and interpersonal control, at the expense of flexibility, openness, and efficiency, beginning by early adulthood and present in a variety of contexts, as indicated by 4 or more of the following:

(1) Is preoccupied with details, rules, lists, order, organization, or schedules to the extent that the major point of the activity is lost.

Has anyone ever told you that you spend too much time making lists and schedules of what you need to do? Do you think you do?

When you have a task to do, do you often spend so much time getting organized that you have trouble getting the job done?

When you are working on something, do you often spend so much time on small details that you lose sight of the main thing you were trying to do?

IF YES: Examples.

(2) Shows perfectionism that interferes with task completion (e.g., is unable to complete a project because his or her own overly strict standards are not met).

Would you say that you are a perfectionist?
Would others?

IF YES TO EITHER: How often do your high standards keep you from getting projects completed on time?

(3) Is excessively devoted to work and productivity to the exclusion of leisure activities and friendships (not accounted for by obvious economic necessity).

Would you call yourself a workaholic?
Have others said this about you?
IF YES TO EITHER: Do you spend so much time working that you have little time for family activities, friendships, or entertainment?
What about vacations?

Is it hard for you to enjoy a vacation because you're worried about getting behind in your work?
Do you usually take work along with you?

How many hours a week do you work?
IF CONSIDERABLE: Why do you work so many hours?
Would you still work that much if you could get the same pay for fewer hours?.

(4) Is overconscientious, scrupulous, and inflexible about matters of morality, ethics, or values (not accounted for by cultural or religious identification).

Do you have a strong sense of moral and ethical values?
IF YES: Do you think you're more concerned about these values than most people you know?
Would you have trouble being friends with someone who disagrees with you on moral or ethical issues?

How often do you worry that you've done something immoral or unethical?

Have other people complained that you are too strict about moral issues?
IF YES: What did they complain about?

(5) Is unable to discard worn-out or worthless objects even when they have no sentimental value.

Some people find it impossible to throw anything away, even when it's old and worn out. Does this sound like you?

IF YES: What kinds of things do you keep?
Why do you keep them?
Do others complain or tease you about the things you save?

(6) Is reluctant to delegate tasks or to work with others unless they submit to exactly his or her way of doing things.

Do you end up doing a lot of jobs yourself because you believe that no one else will do it exactly the way you want it done?

IF YES: Examples?

Do you find yourself taking over other people's responsibilities to make sure that things get done right?

IF YES: Examples.

(7) Adopts a miserly spending style toward self and others: money is viewed as something to be hoarded for future catastrophes.

After you pay your bills, what kinds of things do you like to spend money on?

Are you slow to spend money on yourself?
How about spending money on others?

Some people worry so much about something terrible happening in the future that they save all their money to be prepared for that future catastrophe. Does this sound like you?

IF YES: Tell me about that.

(8) Shows rigidity and stubbornness.

Would other people describe you as being stubborn or set in your ways? What about inflexible or closed-minded?

IF YES TO EITHER: What makes them say that?
Do you agree?

AVOIDANT PERSONALITY DISORDER

Inclusion: at least 4 criteria
Exclusion: None

A pervasive pattern of social inhibition, feelings of inadequacy, and hypersensitivity to negative evaluation, beginning by early adulthood and present in a variety of contexts, as indicated by 4 or more of the following:

(1) Avoids occupational activities that involve significant interpersonal contact, because of fears of criticism, disapproval, or rejection.

Do you try to avoid the kind of work that requires a lot of contact with people or do you enjoy that kind of work?
IF AVOIDS: Why is that?
IF UNCLEAR: Are you afraid that people will criticize or reject you?

Have you ever turned down a job or promotion because it would have required more contact with people?
IF YES: Why is that?

(2) Is unwilling to get involved with people unless certain of being liked.

How often do you avoid getting to know someone because you are worried they may not like you?
IF OFTEN: Has this affected the number of friends you have?

(3) Shows restraint within intimate relationships because of the fear of being shamed or ridiculed.

Even when you're in a close relationship, do you often keep your thoughts and feelings to yourself because you're afraid the other person might put you down?
IF YES: How much has this fear kept you from feeling really comfortable in close relationships?

(4) Is preoccupied with being criticized or rejected in social situations.

In social situations, how much do you worry about being criticized or rejected by other people?

Do you worry about rejection?
IF YES: Tell me about that.
How does this concern affect your behavior?

(5) Is inhibited in new interpersonal situations because of feelings of inadequacy.

Do you have a lot more trouble than most people carrying on a conversation with someone you've just met?
IF YES: What makes it hard?

Do you often feel inadequate in social situations?
IF YES: How much does this get in the way of your meeting new people and making friends?

(6) Views self as socially inept, personally unappealing, or inferior to others.

Do you usually feel like you're not as interesting or fun as other people?

How do you think you relate to people in social situations?
IF POOR: Why do you think that is?

(7) Is unusually reluctant to take personal risks or to engage in any new activities because they may prove embarrassing.

Some people are willing to take some risks or take on new activities, whereas others always play it safe. How would you describe yourself?

How often do you avoid taking chances or trying new activities because you're worried about embarrassing yourself?
IF YES: Examples.

DEPENDENT PERSONALITY DISORDER

Inclusion: at least 5 criteria
Exclusion: None

A pervasive and excessive need to be taken care of that leads to submissive and clinging behavior and fears of separation, beginning by early adulthood and present in a variety of contexts, as indicated by 5 or more of the following:

(1) Has difficulty making everyday decisions without an excessive amount of advice and reassurance from others.

Some people enjoy making decisions and other people prefer to have someone they trust tell them what to do. Which do you prefer?

How much do you look for reassurance or advice about everyday decisions like what to have for lunch or what clothes to buy? Is it difficult for you to make these kinds of decisions on your own?

(2) Needs others to assume responsibility for most major areas of his or her life.

Some people often end up in situations where other people make decisions about important areas of their life. For example, they let someone else decide whether they should take a job, who their friends should be, etc. Does this sound like your life?

IF YES: What keeps you from making decisions on your own?

(3) Has difficulty expressing disagreement with others because of fear of loss of support or approval (NOTE: Do not include realistic fears of retribution).

How hard is it for you to express a different opinion with someone you're close to?

IF HARD: What do you worry might happen if you do?

Do you often pretend to agree with someone so he/she won't reject you or dislike you?

(4) Has difficulty initiating projects or doing things on his or her own (because of a lack of self-confidence in judgment or abilities rather than a lack of motivation or energy).

Do you usually need help from someone else to get started on a project? Is it difficult to get things done on your own?

IF YES TO EITHER: Why is that?
Is it because you don't feel confident in your own abilities?

(5) Goes to excessive lengths to obtain nurturance and support from others, to the point of volunteering to do things that are unpleasant.

Do you bend over backwards to do things for others just so they'll take care of you or support you when you need it?

IF YES: Do you ever volunteer to do unpleasant things for this reason? **IF YES:** Examples.

(6) Feels uncomfortable or helpless when alone, because of exaggerated fears of being unable to care for himself or herself.

How do you usually feel when you're alone?

IF UNCOMFORTABLE:

Are you afraid you won't be able to take care of yourself?

IF YES: In what way?

(7) Urgently seeks another relationship as a source of care and support when a close relationship ends.

What do you do when a close relationship ends?
Would you be desperate to get into another relationship right away, even if it was not the best person for you? **IF YES:** Why is that?

(8) Is unrealistically preoccupied with fears of being left to take care of himself or herself.

How much do you worry about people you depend on leaving you?

IF WORRIES: What has caused your concern?
Are there times you can't stop worrying about this?
Are you worried that you won't be able to take care of yourself?

THE MENTAL STATUS EXAMINATION (MSE)

The mental status examination is analogous to the physical examination. The focus is on current signs, symptoms, affect, behavior, and cognition. Some excellent books and book chapters have been written about the mental status exam; however, students and beginning clinicians usually condense these texts to an outline which they follow when writing up the mental status part of the psychiatric evaluation. On the next page is such an outline.

The outline represents a standardized way of presenting (orally or in writing) the mental status exam. This outline should not be used as a checklist of items to ask of the patients, and should not influence the flow of the psychiatric interview. The best interviewers let the patient do most of the talking (at least at the beginning of the evaluation), and they follow the patient's lead in collecting the mental status exam data base. This differs from the detailed physical exam, in which the order of the exam is often the same for all patients (e.g., start at the head and work downwards).

A good interviewer is not just listening to the content of the patient's speech. He or she is also observing affect and motor behavior, monitoring the amount, flow and quality of speech, and noting whether the connections between words, phrases, and sentences deviates from normal goal directed speech.

Authors vary in how they delineate the sections of the mental status exam. The outline below consists of 10 sections, with multiple components to each. For many of the components, I have included lists of frequently used descriptors. The list is <u>not</u> exhaustive.

A short glossary defining some of the terms that cause the greatest confusion follows the outline. The glossary is arranged in alphabetical order. In parentheses after each term is the section of the mental status examination where the term is used.

MENTAL STATUS EXAMINATION OUTLINE

APPEARANCE:

Age (chronological age and whether person looks this age)
Gender, Race
Body build (thin, obese, cachectic, muscular, frail, medium)
Position (lying, sitting, standing, kneeling)
Posture (rigid, slumped, cross-legged, slouched, comfortable, threatening)
Eye contact
Dress (what individual is wearing, cleanliness, condition of clothes, neatness, appropriateness of garments)
Grooming (malodorous, highly perfumed, dirty, unshaven, kemptness, smelling of alcohol, hairstyle, makeup)
Manner (cooperativeness, guarded, pleasant, evasive, angry, seductive, ingratiating, friendly, inappropriately familiar, glib, hostile, suspicious)
Attentiveness to examiner (disinterested, bored, internally preoccupied, distractible, attentive)
Distinguishing features (scars, tattoos, bandages, blood stains, missing teeth, tobacco stained fingers)
Prominent physical abnormalities (missing limb, jaundice, profuse sweating, goiter, wheezing, coughing)
Emotional facial expression (crying, screaming, tremulous, looking upward as if hearing voices, furrowed brow, calm)
Alertness (alert, drowsy, stupor, comatose)

MOTOR:

Retardation (slowed movements)
Agitation (unable to sit still, wringing hands, restless/bouncing legs, rocking, picking at skin or clothing, pacing)
Abnormal movements (tremor, lip smacking, tongue thrust, mannerisms, grimaces, tics)
Gait (shuffling, broad based, limping, stumbling, festinating)
Catatonia (stupor, excitement, waxy flexibility)

SPEECH:

Rate (slowed, long pauses before answering questions, hesitant, rapid, pressured)
Rhythm (monotonous, stuttering)
Volume (loud, soft, whispered)
Amount (monosyllabic, hypertalkative, mute)
Articulation (clear, mumbled, slurred, dysarthric)
Spontaneity

AFFECT:
- Stability (stable, fixed, labile)
- Range (constricted, full)
- Appropriateness (to content of speech and circumstances)
- Intensity (flat, blunted, exaggerated)
- Type of affect (depressed, sad, happy, euphoric, irritable, anxious, neutral, fearful, angry, apathetic, pleasant)
- Mood (patient's report)

THOUGHT CONTENT:
- Suicidal ideation, death wishes
- Homicidal ideation
- Depressive cognitions (guilt, worthless, hopeless)
- Obsessions, ruminations
- Phobias
- Ideas of reference, paranoid ideation
- Magical ideation
- Delusions
- Overvalued ideas
- Other major themes discussed by patient

THOUGHT PROCESS:
- Associations
- Coherence (coherent, incoherent)
- Logic (logical, illogical)
- Stream (goal directed, circumstantial, tangential, loose, flight of ideas, rambling, word salad)
- Clang associations
- Perseverative
- Neologism
- Blocking
- Attention (distractibility, concentration)

PERCEPTION:
- Hallucinations (auditory, visual, olfactory, gustatory, tactile)
- Illusions
- Depersonalization
- Derealization
- Déjà vu, Jamais vu

INTELLECT: Global evaluation (average, above or below average)

INSIGHT: Awareness of illness

MINI-MENTAL STATE EXAM: (see next page)

MINI-MENTAL STATE EXAMINATION

The Mini-Mental State Examination (MMSE, Folstein et al, 1975) is the most widely used screening evaluation for cognitive impairment. The MMSE has been used to screen for dementia and delirium, grossly quantify the degree of cognitive impairment, and serially measure cognitive changes over time. It should be emphasized that the MMSE is only a screening measure, and it should not be used as the sole criterion for diagnosing dementia.

The MMSE is reprinted on the next two pages. Scores range from 0-30, and values of 23 or less suggest the presence of cognitive impairment. Some authorities recommend that three levels of cognitive impairment be delineated: 24-30 = no cognitive impairment; 18-23 = mild cognitive impairment; and 0-17 = severe cognitive impairment. MMSE scores are correlated with years of education, and the established cutoff points are probably not valid if the patient has less than a ninth grade education.

During the course of a psychiatric evaluation the MMSE can be introduced as follows: "Now I'm going to ask you some questions to test your concentration and memory."

The MMSE has been reprinted with permission from: Folstein MP, Folstein SE, and McHugh PR. "Mini-mental State:" A practical method for grading the cognitive states of patients for the clinician. *Journal of Psychiatric Research*, 1975, 12:189-198.

MINI-MENTAL STATE EXAMINATION (Folstein)

ORIENTATION TO TIME

( ) What year is this? [1 point]
( ) What season of the year is it? [1 point]
( ) What is the month and date? [1 point]
( ) What day of the week is it? [1 point]

ORIENTATION TO PLACE

( ) What is the name of this place? [1 point]
( ) What floor are we on? [1 point]
( ) What city and state are we in? [1 point for each]
( ) What county is this? [1 point]

IMMEDIATE RECALL

( ) I am going to say 3 objects. After I say them I want you to repeat them. They are: "Apple" "Table" "Penny." Now you say them. [1 point for each]. (Interviewer: repeat until all 3 are learned).
Remember what they are because I'm going to ask you to name them again in a few minutes.

ATTENTION (either item)

( ) a) Subtract 7 from 100, then subtract 7 from the answer you got and keep subtracting 7 until I tell you to stop. [1 point each correct answer, maximum 5 points]
b) Spell the word "world" backwards [1 pt each correct letter, max 5]

DELAYED RECALL

( ) What are the 3 words I asked you to remember? [1 point for each].

NAMING

( ) Show patient a pen and watch and ask to name them. [1 pt for each].

REPETITION

( ) Repeat the following sentence exactly as I say it: "No ifs, ands, or buts." [1 point]

3 STAGE COMMAND

( ) Now I want to see how well you follow instructions. I'm going to give you a piece of paper. Take it in your right hand, use both hands to fold it in half, and then put it on the floor. [1 point for each command, max 3 points].

READING

( ) Show the patient page 151 and ask him/her to read what it says at the top silently, to him/herself, and then do what it says. [1 point].

COPYING

( ) Give patient a clean sheet of paper and ask him/her to copy the design printed on page 151. [1 point].

WRITING

( ) On the same sheet of paper, ask patient to write a complete sentence. [1 point]

( ) **Total** (Maximum score = 30)

CLOSE YOUR EYES

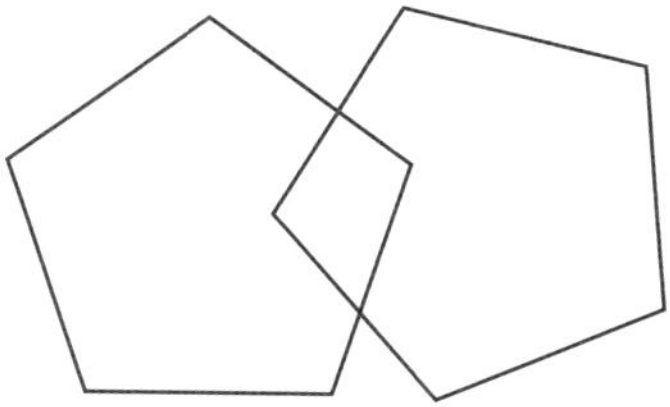

GLOSSARY OF TERMS

Affect The observed emotional state during the evaluation.

1. Blunted affect refers to minimal expression and intensity of emotion. The individual's facial expression varies little. There are few physical gestures of emotion; eye contact is either minimal or the patient seems to stare at the interviewer, and the patient speaks in a monotonous tone with little vocal inflection. The person's face seems to have little muscle tone.

2. Constricted affect refers to a limited range of expressed emotion. The emotion may be intense (severe depression, anger), but there is little variability of expression during the interview.

3. Flat affect is a more severe form of blunted affect with essentially no affective expression. The interviewer may feel as if he or she is conversing with an inanimate object.

4. Inappropriate affect refers to a discordance between the content of speech and the expressed emotion (e.g., laughing while discussing the death of a love one).

5. Labile affect refers to abrupt, rapid, and repeated shifts of type and intensity of emotion.

Alexithymia (affect) Impaired ability to recognize subjective mood state and to describe emotions verbally.

Circumstantiality (thought process) Speech that takes a circuitous route before reaching its goal. Extra, unnecessary, and sometimes tedious details are added. The speaker often needs to be interrupted. However, there is a clearly recognized link between the associations (in contrast to looseness of associations).

Clang Associations (thought process) Speech in which the sounds of words, rather than their meaning, guide the choice of words. Puns and rhymes are characteristic. (e.g., "Where should I lie? If I lie, will I die? Go to the sky, why up high?")

Delusion (thought content) A fixed, false belief that is not shared with members of the individual's culture or religion. The distinction between a delusional and a false nondelusional idea is not always clearcut. For example, a clinically depressed president of a corporation who feels like a failure and a disappointment to her family and friends would usually not be considered delusional unless she claimed to be poverty stricken (despite a sizable bank account), or responsible for causing tragic events to which he or she has no connection. The obsessions of some individuals with obsessive compulsive disorder are firmly held, and only after considerable discussion do they acknowledge that the belief may be incorrect. Underweight anorexics may incorrectly believe they are fat, yet are not considered delusional. Delusions fall into one of the following 14 categories:

1. Delusion of control. Delusional belief that one's actions, behavior, or feelings are not under personal control or own doing, but are imposed by an external force. The essential requirement is that the individual believes his will, thoughts or feelings have been replaced by something external. (e.g., "The spirit of my dead father is inside me and controls me.")

2. Delusion of guilt or sin. Delusional belief of responsibility for tragedy or disaster to which there is no personal connection. (e.g., "The Persian Gulf war was my fault.") Delusional belief of having done something terrible and now must face deserved retribution or punishment.

3. Delusion of grandiosity. Delusional belief of special power, talent, abilities, or identity. (e.g., Individuals who believe they are Christ, an apostle, Hitler, Elvis, etc. Patient believed he was responsible for the Camp David accord between Israel and Egypt, and now was needed in the Middle East to help settle the Palestinian problem.)

4. Delusion of jealousy. With little or no evidence, the person believes one's sexual partner is unfaithful. The person often goes to great effort to prove the existence of the affair. (e.g., A patient attempted to remain awake all night to catch his wife sneaking out of the house. He attached a string from her toe to his. He asserted that after he fell asleep at approximately 4 a.m., his wife slipped off the string, left the house to participate in an orgy, and returned to reattach the string before he awakened. The patient was referred to psychiatry after he brought his wife's panties to the OB-GYN department requesting an examination and analysis of semen residue.)

5. Delusion of mind reading. Delusional belief that people can read one's mind or know one's thoughts. This does not include sensing what a person is thinking by body language or facial expression. It also differs from thought broadcasting (see below), in that the patient does not believe that his thoughts are heard by others.

6. Delusion of persecution. Delusional belief that one is in danger, being followed or monitored, harassed, or conspired against. This may involve government agencies (FBI, police), criminal groups (the mob, mafia, drug dealers), neighbors, coworkers, and even family.

7. Delusion of reference. Delusional belief that ordinary, insignificant comments, objects, or events refer to or have special meaning for the patient. (e.g., Patient believed that songs on the radio had subliminal messages intended specifically for him.)

8. Delusion of replacement. Delusional belief that someone important to the patient (e.g., family member, spouse) has been replaced by a double. Also called Doppelganger.

9. Erotomania. Delusional belief that one is loved, perhaps secretly, by another person. Usually the other person is of higher status than the patient.

10. Nihilistic delusion. Delusional belief that the person, a part of the person's body, or the world does not exist. (e.g., "Aliens took my brain out of my head and put it in the drawer of the desk. I no longer have a brain.")

11. Somatic delusion. Delusional belief that one's body is diseased or changed. (e.g., A depressed man with constipation believed he had colon cancer despite a negative GI work-up. Another male patient believed he was pregnant.)

12. Thought broadcasting. Delusional belief that as thoughts occur they escape from the person's head and can be heard by others. The patient may or may not also hear his thoughts aloud. (e.g., A patient believed that the FBI was tape recording his thoughts, even though he wasn't speaking.)

13. Thought insertion. Delusional belief that thoughts are not one's own, but have been placed there by some person, group, or force from the outside. (e.g., During an interview the patient uttered an obscenity, turned towards a group of patients behind him, and emphatically said to the interviewer that they put that word into his head because he never curses.)

14. Thought withdrawal. Delusional belief that one's thoughts have been removed or taken away by someone or something from the outside.

Déjà vu (perception) The feeling that one has already experienced a particular moment or event before.

Depersonalization (perception) An altered sense of one's physical being. Includes feeling outside of one's body, physically cut off or distanced from people, floating, observing oneself from a distance, like one is in a dream, or that one's body is physically changed in shape or size.

Derealization (perception) A sense that one's environment has changed and is different than the way it had been before, though the individual cannot identify tangible elements of change.

Distractibility (thought process) Attention to the interviewer is easily disrupted by unimportant external stimuli.

Flight of Ideas (thought process) Rapid speech with abrupt changes from topic to topic usually based on understandable links between the topics, distracting external stimuli, or plays on words. When severe, the link between the associations may be so obscure that loose associations or incoherence may also be present (see definitions below).

Hallucinations (perception) A sensory perception in the absence of an actual external stimulus. They can occur in any sensory system of the body: sight, hearing, taste, smell, and touch.

1. Auditory hallucination. Usually refers to hearing voices, but also can refer to hearing noises, sounds, music, etc.

2. Hypnogogic hallucination. Occurs when an individual is falling asleep and is considered a pseudo-hallucination. It has significance only for the diagnosis of abnormal sleep states, and is not indicative of psychopathology.

3. Hypnopompic hallucination. Is analogous to a hypnogogic hallucination, except it occurs upon awakening.

4. Olfactory hallucination. A hallucination involving smell. Of note, the belief that one has a noxious or peculiar body odor is not a hallucination unless the person also smells it.

5. Tactile hallucination. A hallucination involving the sense of touch.

6. Visual hallucination. Usually refers to seeing people or animals, but also can refer to seeing shapes, colors, flashes of light, etc.

Idea of Reference (thought content) Similar to a delusion of reference except the person questions the reality of the belief. (e.g., A patient wondered whether everyone on the bus was talking about him, but knew this was unlikely to be true.)

Illogical Thinking (thought process) Thinking that contains clear internal contradictions, or in which conclusions are reached which make no logical sense. (e.g., "My mother died before I was born.")

Illusion (perception) A misperception of a real external stimulus. This is distinguished from a hallucination which is the perception of a non-existent external stimulus. (e.g., Misinterpretation of shadows as people, or noises as people's voices.)

Jamais Vu (perception) The feeling of unfamiliarity with familiar situations.

Incoherence (thought process) Incomprehensible speech due to disruption of logical or meaningful connection between words or phrases, many incomplete sentences, idiosyncratic use of words, and distorted grammar.

Loose Association (thought process) Speech characterized by a disruption of logical or meaningful connection between the ideas and thoughts in the sequence. Sometimes there is an oblique association between ideas, sometimes there is no association at all. The individual is unaware of the lack of connectedness between the thoughts. Often the interviewer will be left wondering what the patient just said.

Magical Thinking (thought content) The belief that thinking something will cause it to occur. This is normal in children (e.g., children avoiding stepping on a sidewalk crack so they won't "break their mother's back").

Mood (affect) The sustained emotion experience and reported by an individual. This contrasts to affect, which is the emotional tone perceived by an observer.

Neologism (thought process) A new word, distortion of words, or condensed combination of words created by the patient and which has a specific meaning to the patient. (e.g., "I futiligated the rocket to outer space.")

Nonsequitur (thought process) A response that does not follow from the question asked. Often used by politicians. (e.g., "Where were you born?" "I'm not sure if that's the way it's always been or not.")

Overvalued Idea (thought content) A relatively firmly held false belief that is not shared with members of the individual's culture or religion, but which is not maintained with delusional intensity. (e.g., A patient who is concerned about getting AIDS from a public toilet seat acknowledges he may be wrong but still wants an HIV blood test.)

Perseveration (thought process) Repetition of the same word, phrase, or idea in response to different questions. This does not include the use of filler words such as "you know," "like," or "I mean." (e.g., That's my story. Things happen and this is how my story unfolded. My story isn't a very happy one, and I hope my story for the future will be better.)

Preoccupation (thought process) Mental absorption in a particular topic or concern.

Pressured Speech (speech) Rapid, continuous speech that is difficult to interrupt.

Psychosis A severe mental disturbance indicating gross impairment in reality testing. Manifestations of psychosis include delusions, hallucinations, looseness of associations, grossly disorganized and bizarre speech or behavior.

Rambling (thought process) Speech that is fragmented, without goal, and usually associated with intoxication.

Tangentiality (thought process) Speech that talks past the point and never reaches the goal of answering the question. Similar to circumstantial speech, but in contrast to loose associations, there is a clearly recognized link between associations. In contrast to circumstantial speech, the goal is never reached.

Thought Blocking (thought process) A sudden interruption in the spontaneous flow of speech associated with the person saying that his mind went blank. Upon questioning, after a period of silence, the individual states he cannot recall what he was thinking about.

Thought Disorder (thought process) Also referred to as formal thought disorder. A generic term that refers to abnormalities in the form of thought in contrast to the content of thought.

Word Salad (thought process) Speech that is incomprehensible and incoherent because of a lack of logical and meaningful connection between words. It represents the extreme form of looseness of associations.

CURRENT PSYCHOSOCIAL FUNCTIONING

Employment

Do you work?

IF NO: Why didn't you work this past week?

IF YES:

What kind of work do you do?
How many hours per week do you work?
Did you miss any time from work during the past week?

IF YES: How much time did you miss?
For what reason?

Did you have any problems on the job during the past week?

IF YES: Like what?

Does anyone evaluate your performance at work?

IF YES: Who?

IF YES TO EITHER:

What do they look at to determine whether you're doing a good job?
What kind of evaluations have you gotten?
What do <u>you</u> look at to determine if you're doing a good job?
How well did you do your job during the past week?
Could you give me some examples?

IF NO TO BOTH:

What do <u>you</u> look at to determine if you're doing a good job?
How well did you do your job during the past week?
Could you give me some examples?

IF NOT ALREADY CLEAR FROM ABOVE:

In what way did your (PATIENT DESCRIPTION OF HEALTH PROBLEM) affect your job during the past week?
Because of your (HEALTH PROBLEM), were there things you didn't get done at work?

IF YES: Like what?

Did your (HEALTH PROBLEM) cause problems concentrating at work?
Did you work as efficiently as usual?

IF NO: Describe that for me.

Household work

What responsibilities do you have in your household?
Do you do any cleaning? Laundry? Cooking? Shopping?
House repairs or yard work?
Take care of any kids or older or disabled family members?
Run errands? Pay the bills?
Is there anything else that you do to keep your household running?

During this past week how well have you been keeping up with your household responsibilities?
Are there any things you usually do that you didn't get done this past week?
IF YES: What kept you from (TASK)?
Were there days you didn't get anything done?
IF YES: How many days were like that?

Did you have any difficulty doing your household chores?
IF YES: Like what?
How would you rate your performance of household chores for the past week?

IF NOT ALREADY CLEAR FROM ABOVE:
In what way did your (HEALTH PROBLEM) affect your (SPECIFIC CHORES)?
Because of (HEALTH PROBLEM), were there things you didn't get done?
IF YES: Like what?
Were there things you didn't do as well as usual?
IF YES: Like what?

Schoolwork

Do you go to school or take any classes?
IF YES: Are you a full-time student?
IF NO: How many classes do you take?

*****ASK THE FOLLOWING IF AT LEAST A HALF-TIME STUDENT*****

Did you miss or skip any classes this past week?
IF YES: How many? For what reason?

Were you given any assignments, homework, or tests this past week?
IF YES: How did you do?
IF UNSURE: How do you think you did? (How do you usually do?)
How have your study habits been this past week?

IF EVIDENCE OF IMPAIRED FUNCTIONING:

Were there days you didn't get anything done? That is, you couldn't go to classes or you couldn't do any homework or studying?

IF YES: How many days were like that?

IF NOT ALREADY CLEAR FROM ABOVE:
How did your (HEALTH PROBLEM) specifically affect your schoolwork this past week?
Did your (HEALTH PROBLEM) cause problems concentrating?
Did you work as efficiently as usual?
IF NOT: Describe that for me.

Relationships with husband, wife, boyfriend, girlfriend, or lover

---

Are you married?
IF YES: How would you describe your marriage?
How close a relationship do you and your spouse usually have?
How were things this past week?
Did you have any arguments or disagreements this past week?
IF YES: How often did you argue?
For how long did you stay angry at each other?
Were you able to work out your problems?

IF NO: Do you have a boyfriend or girlfriend or lover?
IF YES: How long have you been going with him/her?
Do you live together?
How close is the relationship?
How have you gotten along this past week?
Did you have any arguments or disagreements?
IF YES: How often did you argue?
For how long did you stay angry?
Were you able to work out your problems?

IF NOT ALREADY CLEAR FROM ABOVE:
How did your (HEALTH PROBLEM) affect your relationship?
Did it affect your closeness?
Have you been more withdrawn?
Did you argue more or less?

Relationships with other family members

Who is in your immediate family? Your extended family? Do you have in-laws? Grandparents? Grandchildren? Any other family?

Are your parents still alive?

IF YES: Are you close?
How do you get along with them?
Did you see, speak, or text to them this past week?
Did you have any arguments or disagreements this past week?

IF YES: How often did you argue?
For how long did you stay angry at each other?

Do you have any brothers or sisters?

IF YES: Are you close?
How do you get along with them?
Did you see, speak, or text to them this past week?
How have you gotten along with them this past week?
Did you have any arguments or disagreements this past week?

IF YES: How often did you argue?
For how long did you stay angry at each other?

Do you have any children?

IF YES: Are you close?
How do you get along with them?
Did you see, speak, or text to them this past week?
How have you gotten along with them this past week?
Did you have any arguments or disagreements this past week?

IF YES: How often did you argue?
For how long did you stay angry at each other?

Are there family members that you avoid seeing because of serious problems or trouble getting along?

IF NOT ALREADY CLEAR:

How has your [HEALTH PROBLEM] affected your relationships with your family?
Did it affect your closeness with anyone?
Have you been more withdrawn?
Did you argue more or less with anyone?

Relationships with friends

Not counting your family members, do you have any close friends you can confide in about a personal matter?

IF YES: How many close friends do you have?
How often do you usually see or speak or text to them?
What about this past week?
How have you been getting along with them over the past week?
Any arguments or disagreements?
How strong are the ties between you?

IF NO: How many people do you know that you wouldn't necessarily confide in, but whom you would consider friends?

IF ONE OR MORE:
How often do you usually see or speak or text to them?
What about this past week?
How have you been getting along with your friends over the past week?
Any arguments or disagreements?
How strong are the ties between you?

IF NOT ALREADY CLEAR:
How did your (HEALTH PROBLEM) affect your relationship with your friends?
Did it affect your closeness with anyone?
Have you been more withdrawn?
Did you argue more or less with anyone because of your (HEALTH PROBLEM)?

Recreation

What kinds of leisure or recreational activities do you enjoy?
Do you have any hobbies?
(Are there any activities [outside of work] that you do regularly or occasionally?)
What did you do for fun this past week?

What about: reading? watching or playing sports?
participating in community groups?
exercising? gardening?
going to the movies, plays or concerts?
crafts? watching television? computer games?
listening to or playing music?
going to church, synagogue or temple?
hobbies? parties?

How often did you (ACTIVITY MENTIONED ABOVE)?

How much did you enjoy (ACTIVITY)?

How much did your (HEALTH PROBLEM) affect your participation in leisure, recreational and fun activities?

How much did your (HEALTH PROBLEM) affect your enjoyment of the things you did?

General satisfaction with life

We've reviewed several areas of your life – work, housework, relationships with family and friends, and leisure. The last thing I'd like to ask you about is your level of satisfaction with your life. Considering all the different areas of your life, how satisfied overall have you felt about your life during the past week?

IF GENERALLY SATISFIED:
Are you satisfied with all areas of your life?
IF NO: Which areas are you dissatisfied with?
How dissatisfied are you?
IF YES: Any dissatisfaction in any areas?
IF YES: Which ones?
How dissatisfied are you?

IF GENERALLY DISSATISFIED:
Are you dissatisfied with all areas of your life?
IF NO: Which areas are you satisfied with?
How satisfied are you?
IF YES: Any satisfaction in any area?
IF YES: Which ones?
How satisfied are you?

ORDERING INFORMATION

Title: Interview Guide for Evaluating DSM-5-TR Psychiatric Disorders and the Mental Status Examination (ISBN: 978-0-9633821-2-2)

PRICE LIST

# copies	Cost
1-4	$14.00 (plus $4.00 Shipping & Handling (S/H) = $18.00/copy
5-24	$14.00/copy (S/H included)
25-100 (21% off)	$11.00/copy
> 100	Call for price quote

All orders will be shipped via USPS. Prepayment by check or money order is necessary.

Payable to: Psych Products Press

Mailing address: Psych Products Press
P.O. Box 228
East Greenwich, RI 02818

Phone: (401) 885-6746

Shipping address: ____________________

____

____

____